The Treatment of **PTSD**
with **Chinese Medicine**
—An Integrative Approach

中西医结合治疗创伤后应激障碍

Project Editors: Harry F. Lardner & Zeng Chun
Copy Editor: Chen Xiao-lei
Book Designer: Dai Shan-shan
Cover Designer: Dai Shan-shan
Typesetter: Wei Hong-bo

The Treatment of **PTSD**
with **Chinese Medicine**
—An Integrative Approach

中西医结合治疗创伤后应激障碍

Joe C. Chang, MAOM, Dipl. O.M., L.Ac

Ft. Bliss Restoration & Resilience Center,
William Beaumont Army Medical Center,
U.S.A.

Wang Wei-dong, M.S. TCM

Chief Physician & Professor, Department of TCM Psychology,
Guang'anmen Hospital of China Academy of Chinese Medical Sciences,
Beijing, China

Jiang Yong, Ph.D. TCM

Associate Professor of Chinese Medicine,
Chengdu University of TCM,
Chengdu, China

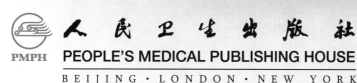

人民卫生出版社
PMPH **PEOPLE'S MEDICAL PUBLISHING HOUSE**

BEIJING · LONDON · NEW YORK

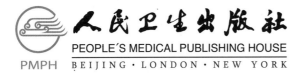

PEOPLE'S MEDICAL PUBLISHING HOUSE

PMPH BEIJING · LONDON · NEW YORK

Website: http://www.pmph.com
Book Title: The Treatment of PTSD with Chinese Medicine—An Integrative Approach
中西医结合治疗创伤后应激障碍

Contact address: No.19, Panjiayuan South Road, Chaoyang District, Beijing 100021, P.R. China, phone/fax: 8610 5978 7399/5978 7338, E-mail: pmph@pmph.com

For text and trade sales, as well as review copy enquiries, please contact PMPH at pmphsales@gmail.com.

First published: 2010
ISBN: 978 - 7 - 117 - 12358 - 7/R · 12359

Cataloguing in Publication Data:
A catalog record for this book is available from the CIP-Database China.

Printed in the People's Republic of China

ISBN 978-7-117-12358-7

Contributors

Wang Mi-qu, M.S. TCM
Chief Physician & Professor of TCM Psychology,
Chengdu University of TCM,
Chengdu, China

Wang Fang, M.S. TCM
Attending Physician of TCM Psychology,
Guang'anmen Hospital

Marie Sprague, D.O.
Chief, Consultation-Liaison Psychiatry,
Carl R. Darnall Army Medical Center,
U.S.A.

Lü Xue-yu, M.S. TCM
Department of TCM Psychology,
Guang'anmen Hospital

Lü Meng-han, M.S. TCM
Department of TCM Psychology,
Guang'anmen Hospital

Wang Hong-zhan, M.S. TCM
Department of TCM Psychology,
Guang'anmen Hospital

Zhao Qiong, Ph.D. TCM
Associate Professor of Chinese Medicine,
Chengdu University of TCM

Hong Lan, MD
Attending Physician, Department
of TCM Psychology, Guang'anmen
Hospital

Hu Yong-dong, M.S.
Associate Chief Physician, Department
of TCM Psychology, Guang'anmen
Hospital

Wang Cai-feng, M.S. TCM
Associate Chief Physician,
Department of Psychosomatic Medicine,
Guang'anmen Hospital

Liu Yan-jiao, Ph.D. TCM
Chief Physician, Department of
TCM Psychology, Guang'anmen
Hospital

Guo Rong-juan, Ph.D. TCM
Chief Physician, Department of
Neurology, Dongfang Hospital of Beijing
University of Chinese Medicine

Zhao Yang
Attending Physician, Department
of TCM Psychology, Guang'anmen
Hospital

Lin Ying-na, M.S. TCM
Department of TCM Psychology,
Guang'anmen Hospital

Sharon J. Wesch, Ph. D
Clinical Psychologist,
Radiant Heart Healing, U.S.A.

Meredith St. John, BA, MAc
Academic Dean, New England School of
Acupuncture

Lisa Conboy, MA, MS, ScD
Co-Research Director, New England
School of Acupuncture

Translated by

Jing Meng, M.S. TCM   **Zheng Qi**

World Federation of Chinese Medicine Societies

About the Authors

Joe C. Chang, MAOM, Dipl. O.M., L.Ac.

Joe Chang is the first acupuncturist in the United States to specialize in the treatment of post-deployment soldiers diagnosed with post-traumatic stress disorder. He has served as an acupuncturist and researcher for the Integrative PTSD Treatment Program at the Ft. Bliss Restoration & Resilience Center at the William Beaumont Army Medical Center, and is a current member of the Military Acupuncture Society.

Dr. Wang Wei-dong, M.S. TCM

Dr. Wang serves as Chief Physician, professor, and director of the TCM Psychology Department at Guang'anmen Hospital affiliated with the China Academy of Chinese Medical Sciences. While engaged in the theoretical and clinical research of TCM psychology for many years, he also specializes in the clinical application of hypnosis for the treatment of depression, anxiety, and PTSD.

Dr. Jiang Yong, Ph.D. TCM

Dr. Jiang is an Associate Professor at the Chengdu University of TCM, where she has remained engaged in research for nearly 10 years. Having authored the textbook, *TCM Behavioral Medicine*, she is now considered to be China's foremost specialist in this emerging branch of Chinese medicine.

Foreword

I first met Joe Chang at the United States' largest Army installation in Fort Hood, Texas while seeking acupuncture for a war-related injury that had evolved into CRPS (Complex Regional Pain Syndrome, also known as RSD or Reflex Sympathetic Dystrophy). Despite working for only a few months at Fort Hood, Joe had already become legendary for his skills as an acupuncturist, especially in the treatment of Post Traumatic Stress Disorder (PTSD). He initially began treating PTSD with acupuncture in April of 2008 at the first Department of Defense-approved program at the Ft. Bliss Restoration & Resilience Center, thus being the only provider to have incorporated Chinese Medicine into the treatment milieu for combat-related psychological disorders in both pilot programs. Joe is a main contributing author to this textbook, and he primarily treats PTSD patients here at our base. Having myself treated close to 9000 patients with PTSD, I realized long ago that there was something lacking in the Western approach. This book can certainly help to fill in the missing pieces.

For Eastern traditionalists, most of the topics covered in this book will not be new, but their application in the treatment of PTSD will be. For Western psychiatric clinicians who are reading this book, the basic biology and psychology of PTSD as discussed here will reflect the most current view; however, the use of energy medicine as a means of treatment will most likely be unfamiliar since modern psychiatry has only just begun to consider Eastern treatment modalities. As more and more soldiers from various countries are becoming afflicted with this disabling disorder, it has become clear that our standard approaches to medication and talk therapy, although beneficial, usually are not effective enough to achieve complete remission.

The groundbreaking initiatives undertaken by the Department of Defense are on the rise, thus making this book's content relevant and applicable for both Eastern and Western medical practitioners. We ask practitioners of both traditions to maintain an open mind regarding the content and modalities contained within these pages, while also remembering to avoid any temptation to perform any treatment method outside their scope of practice. Lastly, we would like to offer our gratitude to those men, women and children who have sacrificed so much in service of their respective countries. We truly hope that the material contained in this book will offer clinical insight and higher success rates in the treatment of PTSD.

Marie Sprague, D.O.
MAJ, MC
Chief, Consultation-Liaison Psychiatry
Carl R. Darnall Army Medical Center
Fort Hood, Texas
October, 2009

Preface

Post-Traumatic Stress Disorder (PTSD) is a multi-faceted disorder that affects a person at all levels of the body, mind, and spirit; it has also become clear to us that an integrative approach is required in order to fully heal those afflicted. PTSD involves dysfunctions of the channel system, also causing energetic imbalances within the body that standard Western treatment approaches cannot fully address. However, the traditional Chinese medical approach also cannot mend a disorder that involves such a variety of biological dysfunctions (i.e., abnormal levels of cortisol and serotonin). To truly make an impact on such a multi-dimensional disorder that touches on so many different aspects, we recommend a synergistic approach that combines both Chinese Medicine and Western protocols.

This book is a result of a truly international collaboration. Much of the material here originates with the work of an acupuncturist who has treated thousands of patients at two integrative PTSD programs for the U.S. Army. The clinical insights gleaned from these encounters are also supplemented by generous contributions from a team of selected experts from the Guang'anmen Hospital in Beijing, and the Chengdu University of Traditional Chinese Medicine.

This book first highlights the causes of PTSD from a Western medical perspective: epidemiology, symptoms, neuro-chemical alterations, physiological changes and current Western treatments. The causes of PTSD are then described in Chinese medical terms, followed by TCM pattern differentiation and treatment of the acute and chronic phases. Chinese medicinal formulas and acupoints are discussed according to each presenting pattern (i.e. spleen and heart deficiency), but most importantly, this book provides an overview of the integrative approach used at the Fort Bliss Restoration & Resilience Center. In this program, cognitive-behavioral and cathartic psychotherapies are combined with acupuncture, Reiki, therapeutic massage, meditation, expressive art therapy and yoga. Representative case studies are also examined here.

Acknowledgements

Writing and publishing this book would have been impossible without the keen insight of my editors at PMPH in Beijing, China. Thank you for your faith in my idea and for putting up with my stubborn nature. I also offer my gratitude to my father, my mentor in Chinese Medicine for the past twenty years. I can still remember beginning to follow him around at the age of six, when he always took the time to indulge my endless curiosity.

Thanks to Dr. Fortunato for taking a chance on an acupuncturist from San Antonio; to you I owe my entire career, and I am forever grateful. Thanks to Dr. Wesch and to Dr. Thomas for shaping my knowledge of psychology, and to Dr. Sprague for your example of brilliance and courage; you have shown me what it takes to be a well-rounded physician. I am especially grateful to Bob for showing me what selflessness truly exemplifies, and to my friends Kathy, Adon, Albert, and Rachel for being there for me through every trial and tribulation. Thank you to Naila and Tom for your loving and caring advice, and for your constant willingness to lend a helping hand.

Finally, this book is for Corina. You are the love of my life, always the ray of light that guides my path.

Joe C. Chang, MAOM, Dipl. O.M., L.Ac.
October, 2009

Introduction

It has been my great fortune to work with many veterans in treatment at two integrative PTSD programs here in the United States. As an acupuncturist, it is also clear to me that these veterans are truly resilient. Even after all of the pain caused by shrapnel still lodged in their bodies, the anguish of lost comrades, nightmares, countless years spent away from their families, panic attacks, and the depression that these veterans have endured, they continue to return here to heal their wounds and to recapture their lost souls.

But what we have to realize is that it takes more than just standard treatment methods to treat these wounded warriors. It takes more than just medication, and it takes more than individual counseling; to heal our combat veterans as a collective whole, this requires a truly integrative approach. Acupuncture is an effective modality, even more effective when applied in conjunction with conventional methods of cognitive behavioral therapy. Sergeants and privates alike seek relief from the constant state of hyperarousal that incessantly debilitates their lives; most are also frequented with panic attacks, memory loss, lack of sleep, and hypervigilance. Being on ten different medications for their post-concussion syndrome headaches, for their traumatic brain injuries, for their back and knee pains, for their anxiety and panic attacks, for their insomnia, nightmares and other symptoms of PTSD is not what these veterans had envisioned for the rest of their lives. This is certainly no way to live.

One private who drove a tank told me his story, recounting the countless number explosions that he had endured, and one particularly traumatic event that eventually caused him to be medically evacuated to a military treatment facility. The weapon that split his Bradley tank in half also caused his back to become broken in three places, and his neck vertebrae had been fused together. He was constantly agitated from back and neck pain even though Fentanyl was prescribed, and he was also diagnosed with post-traumatic stress disorder. He told me that he also felt like an addict, a pathetic person that cannot live without a quick fix; so everyday he simply ate, slept, and popped his medication.

His life radically changed, however, when he entered our integrative PTSD program. He learned to control his emotions through tai-chi and meditation, and through counseling he was able to process his traumatic experience and impaired cognition of the event. Acupuncture treatments also helped him greatly with his anxiety and back pain. When he graduated the program, he took a bag filled with medication, dropped it off at his physician's desk, and said, "Here is your poison; I am not taking these anymore." He is now a tai-chi instructor here at our integrative PTSD program, now helping many others who have experienced similar traumatic events in military service.

Contents

Chapter 1
Historical Perspectives on PTSD

Both modern and ancient Chinese perspectives of PTSD were clearly documented during their respective periods of time. From a Western perspective, PTSD can be traced back to the American Civil War when a severe nervous condition was recognized in some veterans. Fifty years later, during World War I, physicians coined the term "shell shock" to describe mental and physical symptoms of veterans who had experienced life-threatening events.

From the Chinese historical perspective, the symptoms of PTSD were first documented in the *The Yellow Emperor's Inner Classic* (*Huáng Dì Nèi Jīng*) and also in later works such as *The Classic of Difficult Issues* (*Nàn Jīng*). Although the term PTSD did not exist at that time, both texts contain a number of documented cases of patients with the related symptoms of depression, agitation, anxiety, and loss of appetite.

WESTERN HISTORICAL PERSPECTIVE

Post-Traumatic Stress Disorder (PTSD) is no stranger to health care literature, although it has gone by many names in the last 300 years. In the book titled "Trauma and Recovery" written by a Harvard professor Dr. Judith Herman, she stated, "Clear documentation of the condition dates back to the American Civil War, when a nervous disorder known as Da Costa's Syndrome was recognized in some veterans. Fifty years later, physicians in Great Britain coined the term "shell shock" to describe the physical and mental effects suffered by soldiers who were subjected to or witnessed life-threatening experiences during World War I." Swiss military physicians in 1678 identified a group of symptoms that correlate with the modern Diagnostic and Statistical Manual of Mental Disorders which is often used to diagnose psychiatric disorders. The Swiss physicians described the clusters of symptoms as "nostalgia". These symptoms included melancholy, insomnia, loss of appetite, anxiety, palpitations, and stupor. At about the same time period, German physicians described the same clusters of symptoms as homesickness (*heimweh*).

History also tells us that among the Egyptians, Romans, and Greeks, men began showing signs of combat stress during the atrocities of war. The Greek historian Herodotus wrote of the Athenian warriors during the battle of Marathon, "Warriors went permanently blind when the soldier next to him was killed." Herodotus also wrote that the Spartan commander Leonidas during the battle of Thermoplyae Pass recognized symptoms of combat stress in his warriors. Herodotus wrote, "They had no heart for the fight and were unwilling to take their share of danger."

Under conditions of unremitting exposure to the horrors of trench warfare, men began to break down in shocking numbers. Dr. Herman wrote, "Confined and rendered helpless, subjected to constant threat of annihilation, and forced to witness the mutilation and death of their comrades without hope of any reprieve, many soldiers began to act like hysterical women. They screamed and wept uncontrollably. They froze and could not move. They became mute and unresponsive. They lost their memory and their capacity to feel."

During the First World War, of the two million men that fought overseas, 159,000 soldiers were out of action for psychiatric problems. In the Second World War, in the U.S. Army alone, 504,000 men were out of action with psychiatric problems. In the Korean War, of the 5.7 million U.S. troops that were deployed, mental health casualties were reported to be at 37 per 1,000. In Vietnam, 3.4 million served with a reported mental health casualty rate of 12 per 1,000. In the current War On Terror, of the 1.64 million troops that have been deployed to Afghanistan and Iraq, approximately 300,000 individuals suffer from PTSD or major depression.

Advanced treatment and diagnosis of PTSD started during the Vietnam War. It was at this time that the U.S. government created a more formal infrastructure in the medical system for the treatment of PTSD. It was also at this time that the nation started to express concerns for the mental health of our Vietnam veterans and in 1970, Congress conducted the first hearing to address this medical condition.

One unique feature of the current War On Terror that may be influencing the rates of mental health injuries is the extended deployments that Iraq and Afghanistan veterans have to endure. According to the Rand study titled "Invisible Wounds of War", military deployments during the Iraq and Afghanistan campaigns has increased exponentially, where troops are seeing more frequent deployments accompanied with shorter periods of rest. Under current conditions, mental health casualties will certainly rise. Two American psychiatrists during the Second World

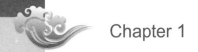

War, J.W. Appel and G.W. Beebe concluded that 200-240 days in combat would suffice to break even the strongest soldier. Each moment of combat imposes a strain so great that men will break down in direct relation to the intensity and duration of their exposure.

ANCIENT CHINESE PERSPECTIVES

Chinese Medical Psychology—Warring States Period to Han & Tang Dynasties

During the Warring States Period, there were various schools of thought regarding health preservation through the avoiding of over-indulgences and through control of one's desires; these ideas can be considered as the beginning of TCM psychotherapy. The *Yellow Emperor's Inner Classic*, the earliest Chinese medical text, also contains aspects of TCM psychology. One such aspect includes the fundamental concept that unless the spirit is stable and well-regulated, physical disease cannot be cured. Thus, TCM treatments should always begin with regulation of the spirit.

It was during this time period that the great scholars and physicians of the time began to emphasize psychological balance and regulation. During the Pre-Qin Period, Lao-tzu and Confucius both advocated controlling one's passions and desires in order to prolong life. Later Qin and Han Dynasty physicians Zhang Zhong-jing and Hua Tuo also gave priority to mental health by advocating both physical exercise and self-cultivation practices.

Jin and Yuan Dynasties

During this period, social unrest in Chinese society led to the formation of different schools of thought, and it was during this period that psychotherapeutic methods were beginning to be applied more extensively. Inspired by the ancient medical classics, four great physicians from this period went on to form different schools of thought.

Physician Liu Wan-su focused on the etiology of emotion, and he also put forward the view that overacting of the five minds can result in excessive internal heat. He stated that "emotions corresponding with the five *zang* organs are anger, joy, anxiety, thinking, and fear."

Overacting of the five minds can damage their corresponding *zang* organs with excessive heat, which also correlates the relationship between psychological states and physical disease. In his opinion, the concept of "the heart governs spirit" also plays a key role in the processes of the five emotions. Even with excessive joy, the end result is the manifestation of internal fire. In the clinical treatment of psychological conditions, clearing heart fire remains as a key treatment principle even today.

In his book *Treatise on the Spleen and Stomach (Pí Wèi Lùn)*, Li Dong-yuan pointed out that the spleen and the stomach can become damaged due to improper diet as well as by environmental factors. He stated that joy, anger, anxiety, and fear can damage upright qi and even exacerbate heart fire, further impairing the upright. In fact, he also stated that sorrow and over-thinking could also cause damage. Regardless of the emotion, the resultant hyperactive internal fire also goes on to impair proper functioning of the spleen and the stomach.

Zhu Dan-xi pointed out that many lifestyle factors can impact one's health, and in his text, *Teachings of [Zhu] Dan-xi (Dān Xī Xīn Fǎ)* he also emphasized psychotherapeutic methods. Fire associated with the five minds results from overacting of the seven emotions, and based on the etiology, he states that these patterns can be treated with psychotherapy instead of herbs or needles. Zhu Dan-xi recommended the use of an antagonistic emotion to treat a current psychological state of disharmony. For example, when a patient is manifesting excess anger, worry and apprehension can be used to counteract that emotion. With excessive joy, anger and worry can be used to counteract that, etc.

In the *Confucians' Duties to Their Parents (Rú Mén Shì Qīn)*, Zhang Cong-zheng summarized the main syndromes related to emotions of anger, joy, sorrow, and fright, also focusing on the methods of using one emotion to counteract another. For example, the language of sorrow is used to treat patients with anger, joy to treat sorrow, fear to treat excessive joy, anger to treat worry and apprehension, and worry and apprehension to counteract fear. Based on the foundation of *The Yellow Emperor's Inner Classic*, Zhang Cong-zheng also discussed the use of desensitization in the treatment of fear or phobias by gradually exposing the patient to the

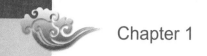

fearful stimuli until it becomes tolerable.

Behavior, Emotion, and Health

Pre-Qin to the *Neijing* Period

During the Spring and Autumn Periods and the Warring States Period, physicians began to focus on the relationships between specific behaviors, health, and disease. Physician Zi Chan stated that "disease is correlated with behaviors, diet, and emotion". Additionally, *Lü's Spring and Autumn* (*Lǔ Shì Chūn Qiū*) also stresses the importance of proper eating habits, and that the over-consumption of fat and alcohol can result in psychological illness.

The Yellow Emperor's Inner Classic discusses the relationship between human behavior and the state of the zang-fu organs and qi and blood, as well as by distinguishing the typical behaviors of different regions and social backgrounds. The role of behavior is also discussed in regards to disease prevention and health preservation, including discussions on personality types, temperaments, five *zang* organs, and the seven emotions. Thus the principles of diagnosis and treatment in *The Yellow Emperor's Inner Classic* can be said to have established the foundation of behavioral-based therapy.

Later on, books such as *Case Records* (*Zhěn Jí*) and the *Treatise on Cold Damage and Miscellaneous Diseases* (*Shāng Hán Zá Bìng Lùn*) also discussed behavioral theory. *Case Records* describes many conditions related to unrestrained sexual activity and excessive alcohol consumption. Zhang Zhong-jing also described the role of certain pathogenic factors that contribute to the development of diseases such as a faulty diet, emotional disorders, alcohol consumption, sexual behavior, and strenuous physical work.

Tang and Song Dynasties—Forming a System

An understanding of the correlation between health, disease, and behavior was further developed after the Qin and Han Dynasties. The *Treatise on the Origins and Manifestations of Various Diseases* (*Zhū Bìng Yuán Hòu Lùn*) states that etiology of disease falls into five distinct categories, and according to the *Classic of Difficult Issues*, important disease factors include behaviors related to diet and labor. Furthermore, specific conditions involving consumptive thirst, jaundice, dysentery, fluid retention, and depressive psychosis are described as mainly caused by improper diet, sexual overindulgence, or improper living conditions. In the *Analects of Bao Pu-zi* (*Bào Pǔ Zǐ*), Ge Hong points out that long-time accumulation of damage to the body caused by emotional disorders, alcohol consumption, improper diet, and excessive labor can lead to an early death.

Throughout the Sui and Tang Dynasties, the understanding of these behavioral factors in disease continued to deepen. Tang Dynasty physician Yang Shang-shan also emphasized that people should control their diet and sexual lifestyle, and in the *Important Formulas Worth a Thousand Gold Pieces* (*Qiān Jīn Yào Fāng*), Sun Si-miao stated "don't eat too much, don't drink too much, don't lift heavy objects, don't over concentrate, don't be fearful, don't laugh too much, don't desire too much, and do not hate others, for all of these behaviors will impact your body".

Two important behavioral theories also emerged after the Song Dynasty. Firstly, in the *Treatise on Diseases, Patterns, and Formulas Related to the Unification of the Three Etiologies* (*Sān Yīn Jí Yī Bìng Zhèng Fāng Lùn*) Chen Wu-ze divides the causative factors of disease into three categories; external factors include cold, heat, wind, and summer-heat, internal factors include joy, anger, worry, and over-thinking, and also other factors which include improper diet and strenuous physical work.

Another other feature of behavioral theory during this period is a greater emphasis on diagnosis according to behaviors and their pathogenic characteristics that lead to disease, including their corresponding treatment and prevention methods. Li Dong-yuan focused on diseases characterized by internal damage, and he also found that improper behaviors in regards to diet, mental stimulation, and physical activities all could lead to spleen-stomach conditions and other disorders. Zhu Dan-xi also discussed lifestyle factors as related to pathomechanisms of damp-heat, frenetic stirring of ministerial fire, and effulgent fire due to yin deficiency.

Chapter 2
Introduction to TCM Psychology

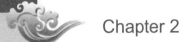

Since the time of Descartes, the predominant Western view of the mind and body includes a distinct separation between the two, and the idea of a "mind-body" connection is tenuous at best. According to the DSM-IV, psychiatry and psychology divide and categorize psychiatric diseases, for example, into anxiety, somatoform, or mood disorders. However, in terms of psychology in Chinese Medicine, there is no distinct separation of the body and mind. The functions of the psyche and physical body are viewed as inseparable, and thus both aspects can be treated together. The body is seen as the material basis for the existence of the mind; as stated in the *Zhōng Yī Jīng Shén Bìng Xué* (Psychiatry of Traditional Chinese Medicine): "Essence, blood, fluids, and humor are the material basis of the spirit."

TCM and Emotion

According to the unified concept of the body and spirit from TCM psychology, all emotional activity is based on the state of qi and blood and the *zang-fu* organs, in fact, emotional changes are also seen as manifestations of *zang-fu* organ function. So, the functional activities of the internal organs will affect the generation and changes of emotion, while emotional change also can affect functional activities of the internal organs. The nature of these emotional changes is dependent upon the coordinated activity of organ function as guided by the heart-spirit. With normal regulation of the heart-spirit, the five *zang* organs are each associated with specific emotional reactions. In any event, the heart is seen as a main component in the etiology of psychological disease. Any blockage or stagnation that affects the functions of heart qi and blood can also result in psychological disease.

Ever since Chen Wu-ze authored *Treatise on Diseases, Patterns, and Formulas Related to the Unification of the Three Etiologies*, Chinese physicians have generally divided the primary cause of disease into three categories: external, internal, and causes neither internal nor external.

Causes of Psychological Disease

External Causes: The Six Environmental Excesses

The six environmental excesses are wind, cold, heat, summer heat, dampness, and dryness. Any of these external evils may lead to the manifestation of pathological symptoms throughout the body. Regarding the external causes of psychological diseases, Tang Dynasty physician Sun Si-miao wrote, "Wind entering the yang channels leads to mania, while wind entering the yin channels leads to withdrawal". However, over the next twelve centuries, Chinese medicine tended to mainly emphasize internal causes and those deemed neither internal nor external as the main etiological factors for psychological conditions.

Neither Internal nor External

Causes neither internal nor external mainly include improper diet, lack of regulation between activity and stillness, and unrestrained sexual behavior.

Improper Diet

In Chinese medicine, there are three main mechanisms that contribute to psychological diseases as associated with an improper diet: malnourishment, heat harassing internally, and blockage and obstruction. In Chinese medical dietary theory, the spleen governs the transformation and transportation of food and fluids within the body, and the heart and spirit both require proper nourishment from the spleen. Therefore, if splenic function becomes impaired by an improper diet, the heart will lack nourishment and the spirit will become disquieted. For example, foods that are high in oil, fat, and sugar tend to damage the spleen, as do chilled, cold-natured, and uncooked foods. Overeating in general can also damage the spleen. Spleen dysfunction leads to impaired transformation of qi and blood, malnourishment of the heart-spirit, and disquietude.

Internal heat harassing the heart is another cause of psychological disease. The over-consumption of hot-natured foods can leads to internal heat that tends to rise upward to harass the heart-spirit. Such foods include peppers, chilies, cinnamon, ginger, black pepper, lamb, beef, and alcoholic beverages.

When the orifices of the heart become blocked, psychological disease can result, and the main pathogenic factors here include phlegm and dampness. As discussed above, fatty meats, oils, and dairy products tend to damage the spleen, where excess phlegm and dampness are produced.

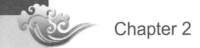

As internal heat causes fluids to congeal, the combining of these internal pathogenic factors can affect the heart and spirit.

Lack of Regulation—Activity and Stillness

Movement can be considered as an activity that consumes qi and blood, where too much activity may exhaust heart qi and deplete yin-blood. When yin becomes damaged, yang qi rises to harass the heart, also affecting the spirit.

On the other hand, too little movement can lead to qi and blood stagnation where qi becomes unable to move blood and fluids properly. Also, food cannot be transformed sufficiently by the spleen, which can result in internal dampness and phlegm accumulation. Thus, lack of movement may also lead to disquieting of the heart.

Unrestrained Sexuality

In Chinese medicine, too much or too little sexual activity can result in psychological disease. The *Treatise on the Spleen and Stomach* states that heart-fire originates from the lower burner, and also that ministerial fire is the fire of the pericardium. In other words, the ministerial fire is rooted in the lower burner and it also connects to the heart in the upper burner. Excessive sexual activity acts to stir up the ministerial fire, also causing yang qi to rise upward. With yang hyperactivity, heat will rise upward and harass the heart.

On the other hand, it is also said that too little sexual activity can be detrimental to the mind, since unfulfilled desires lead to liver qi stagnation. In Chinese medicine theory, the orgasm is described as a release of yang, also associated with yin transformation. Physiologically, the act of ejaculation involves a discharge of qi, so when practiced in moderation, the orgasm acts to promote the free flow of qi.

The Seven Affects

In Chinese Medicine, PTSD is caused primarily by recurrent stimulation of the seven affects: joy, thought, anxiety, sorrow, fear, fright, and anger. Such recurrent stimulation can internally damage three main viscera: the spleen, heart, and liver. The resulting visceral dysfunction also disturbs qi and blood; for example, the liver and spleen have a reciprocal relationship where a dysfunction in one viscus can affect the other. Excessive anger mainly affects the liver, causing qi stagnation and eventually spleen qi deficiency. Persistent liver qi stagnation also leads to the accumulation of internal fire that will damage yin-fluids. Fire tends to have an upward effect that disturbs the heart and disquiets the spirit.

Excessive worry, over-thinking, and anxiety can also damage the spleen and heart, manifesting with insufficiencies of heart-blood and spleen qi. In this case, the heart lacks nourishment and thus the spirit becomes disquieted. With excessive fear and fright, the qi mechanism becomes depressed and stagnant, and when this endures, blood stagnation and the obstruction of the heart vessels will result. (Flaws, 2001)

Recurrent Stimulation

↓

Damaged Viscera

↓

Dysfunction of Qi and Blood

↓

Disturbance of the Heart

The Six Depressions

During the Yuan Dynasty, Zhu Dan-xi formulated the six depressions, which describe stagnations of qi, blood, dampness, phlegm, food, and fire.

Qi depression is mainly a result of unfulfilled desires, which impairs the ability of the liver to govern the free flow of qi. Because post-traumatic stress disorder tends to be construed by the patient as a disorder that is beyond their control, in the same way, qi cannot flow freely. Furthermore, when the desire to feel normal again is not fulfilled, liver qi will become even more stagnant.

Blood depression results from traumatic injury damaging the channels and vessels, from qi stagnation, or from blood deficiency not nourishing the vessels. Qi is the commander of blood, so when the movement of qi is stagnated, there will also be a stagnation of blood. Conversely, blood stagnation and stasis also causes qi depression.

Damp depression involves the accumulation of fluids. One of the functions of qi is to move fluids, so qi stagnation can also lead to dampness accumulation. Over time, dampness accumulation will impede the free flow of qi, and this may also result in depression.

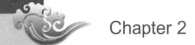

Lingering dampness can congeal to form phlegm, and phlegm also tends to obstruct and hinder the free flow of qi. Phlegm accumulation can aggravate patterns of qi depression by obstructing the free flow of qi.

Food is a material substance that is normally transported and transformed by qi. Overeating can cause qi to become stagnant and depressed, and the free flow of qi becomes impaired.

Yin-Fire and Psychological Diseases

Li Dong-yuan created a disease theory involving yin-fire, which is described as a pathological fire that rises from the middle and lower burners to harass the upper. The heart is located in the upper burner, and is also known as the house of the spirit. Both qi counterflow and heat surging upward can disquiet the heart and spirit. The five main disease mechanisms for yin-fire are spleen deficiency, liver depression, damp-heat, yin-blood deficiency, and stirring of the ministerial fire.

When the spleen becomes weakened, dampness will accumulate in the lower burner and obstruct the free flow of qi. Over time, the accumulated dampness and qi stagnation transform into damp-heat that eventually rises to the upper burner to harass the heart.

With liver depression, the free flow of qi is also impaired, also leading to accumulated heat rising upward to disquiet the heart. The internal heat may also damage the liver and kidneys, causing blood and yin deficiency which cause deficiency heat to rise and disquiet the heart.

The stirring of ministerial fire is caused by excessive mental, verbal, or physical activity. Since the ministerial fire is anchored in the lower burner, its stirring causes the fire to abandon its root. As the ministerial fire stirs upward, it damages and consumes yin-fluids, leaving the lower burner deficient and cold. As stated above, any upward surging of heat can disturb the heart.

Chapter 3
TCM Diagnosis and Treatment

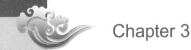

Chapter 3

Even though PTSD is mainly viewed as a psychological maladjustment due to sudden traumatic stimulation, in terms of Traditional Chinese Medicine, PTSD is for the most part treated in the same manner as other somatic diseases. TCM treatments remain based upon the presenting signs and symptoms and pattern differentiation in accordance with physiological changes in the pulse and tongue.

Chinese medicine emphasizes the human-nature inter-relationship, and holds that the environment, society, and the individual function together as an organic whole. Therefore, during the process of TCM therapy, practitioners should focus both on the patient and on the environment around him, particularly the environmental factors that contribute to the abnormal thoughts and behavior. This concept emphasizes social relationships and their overall correlation with behavioral and psychological conditions.

We may notice that the surrounding environment, family members, or friends may actually have a negative impact on the patient. Abnormal psychological behavior in those people related to the patient will worsen their condition; on the other hand, healthy psychological behaviors in people related to the patient will be beneficial, also improving the results of clinical treatment. If PTSD is treated without also considering the patient's surrounding environment, there may be delayed clinical outcomes or the treatment plan may even become completely ineffective.

Furthermore, a comprehensive TCM treatment for PTSD includes a combined treatment approach utilizing both medication and acupuncture. These modalities act to regulate organ function and promote qi and fluid circulation to relieve the symptoms of PTSD, while TCM psychological and behavioral therapies may be applied to correct the abnormal psychological and behavioral issues.

The symptoms of PTSD are complex and interrelated, so TCM psychological or behavioral therapies cannot be utilized as the only treatment modalities. Furthermore, TCM psychological and behavioral therapies do need to be applied concurrently. Generally speaking, a variety of treatment modalities must be applied together in order to achieve satisfactory results.

TCM Patterns and Treatment

In our experience of PTSD cases in the U.S.A., the most common clinical presentations generally involve an excess pattern, with heart and liver channels both affected. Most patients will display anger, frequent panic attacks, anxiety, left arm numbness, heaviness in the chest, and dream-disturbed sleep.

After balancing the liver and the heart channels, signs of an underlying deficiency pattern will emerge, usually involving the spleen and the kidney. Patients will report fatigue, a lack of interest in normal activities, loss of memory, poor digestion and appetite, and lumbar discomfort.

Regarding the excess pattern affecting the liver and heart channel, we believe the autonomic systems are primarily affected. For the spleen and the kidney pattern, the adrenals appear to be most affected.

The TCM patterns and formulas as described below represent a cross-section of typical cases from both China and the United States.

EXCESS PATTERNS

(1) Liver Qi Stagnation
【Signs and Symptoms】
Hyperarousal aggravated by suppressed emotions (i.e., anxiety, over-thinking, anger, and sorrow), mental depression, irritability, unstable mood, distending pain in the chest and hypochondria, frequent hiccups and sighing, poor appetite, insomnia, globus hystericus, and abdominal masses in more serious cases. In females there will be irregular menstruation, dysmenorrhea, distending breast pain and lower abdominal discomfort. The tongue is red with a thin white coating, and the pulse is wiry or slippery.

【Pathomechanism】
The liver governs the regulation of qi, which is also affected by emotions such as fear, anxiety, anger, and sorrow. Qi disharmony and excessive emotion both affect the normal movement of qi within the body; as the liver fails to govern the free movement of qi, other manifestations of liver qi stagnation will appear.

The liver is said to prefer the free flow of qi and also that it is averse to depression. Branches of the liver channel travel along the hypochondriac region, and these pathways also can become obstructed when the liver fails to govern the free flow of qi. Therefore, the clinical manifestations of liver qi stagnation may include pain in the hypochondriac region and frequent sighing along with irritability and a depressed mood.

Furthermore, the normal circulation of body fluids depends on the proper movement of qi. In many cases, liver qi stagnation also leads to the obstructed movement of body fluids, often causing the formation of phlegm. Phlegm that rises along the liver channel divergence to reach the throat can manifest as globus hystericus, where the obstruction of phlegm and qi can also result in goiter. Long-term obstruction leads to patterns of blood stasis and even the formation of masses in the hypochondriac region.

In females, liver qi stagnation can also be viewed in terms of blood movement. The liver not only governs the free flow of qi, but also stores blood and governs the *Chong* and *Ren* channels. Thus liver qi stagnation leads to obstructed blood circulation, disharmony of qi and blood, and impairment the Chong and Ren channels. Impairment of the *Chong* and *Ren* manifests with distending pain in the breasts, dysmenorrhea, and irregular menstruation. The wiry pulse is also an indication of liver qi stagnation.

【Treatment Principle】
Soothe the liver, regulate qi.

【Prescription】
Modified *Chái Hú Shū Gān Sǎn* (Bupleurum Liver-Soothing Powder)

柴胡	*chái hú*	10g	Radix Bupleuri
白芍	*bái sháo*	15g	Radix Paeoniae Alba
川芎	*chuān xiōng*	10g	Rhizoma Chuanxiong
枳壳	*zhǐ qiào*	10g	Fructus Aurantii
香附	*xiāng fù*	10g	Rhizoma Cyperi
陈皮	*chén pí*	10g	Pericarpium Citri Reticulatae
郁金	*yù jīn*	10g	Radix Curcumae
甘草	*gān cǎo*	6g	Radix et Rhizoma Glycyrrhizae

【Formula Analysis】

Chái hú (Radix Bupleuri), *xiāng fù* (Rhizoma Cyperi) and *zhǐ qiào* (Fructus Aurantii) act to soothe the liver, relieve depression, and regulate qi.

Chén pí (Pericarpium Citri Reticulatae) and *yù jīn* (Radix Curcumae) move qi and resolve phlegm.

Chuān xiōng (Rhizoma Chuanxiong), *bái sháo* (Radix Paeoniae Alba) and *gān cǎo* (Radix et Rhizoma Glycyrrhizae) activate blood, relieve pain, and regulate the liver.

【Modifications】

➢ With frequent sighing, add *guā lóu pí* (Pericarpium Trichosanthis) 15g and *xiè bái* (Bulbus Allii Macrostemi) 15g to regulate qi and soothe the chest.

➢ With distending pain in the hypochondriac region, add *yán hú suǒ* (Rhizoma Corydalis) 15g, baked *chuān liàn zǐ* (Fructus Toosendan) 15g, and *fó shǒu* (Fructus Citri Sarcodactylis) 10g to regulate qi and relieve pain.

➢ With localized stabbing pains due to qi stagnation and blood stasis, add *hóng huā* (Flos Carthami) 10g and *táo rén* (Semen Persicae) 10g to move blood and resolve stasis.

➢ With insomnia, add *suān zǎo rén* (Semen Ziziphi Spinosae, baked) 20g to 30g, and *hé huān pí* (Cortex Albiziae) 20g to tranquilize the spirit and soothe the liver.

➢ With anorexia or poor appetite, add *gǔ yá* (Fructus Setariae Germinatus, baked) 20g and *mài yá* (Fructus Hordei Germinatus, baked) 20g to promote digestion and strengthen the stomach.

➢ With distending pain in the hypochondriac region, belching, acid reflux, nausea, and vomiting that is aggravated by fluctuations in mood, add *Píng Wèi Sǎn* (Stomach-Calming Powder) or *Xuán Fù Dài Zhě Tāng* (Inula and Hematite Decoction) to harmonize the stomach and relieve pain.

(2) Liver Depression Transforming into Fire

【Signs and Symptoms】

Hyperarousal, irritability, severe headaches, dizziness, red eyes and red complexion, tinnitus, a bitter taste in the mouth, dry throat, thirst with a preference for cold water, burning pain in the hypochondriac region,

insomnia, nightmares, dry stools, and dark yellow urine. The tongue is red with a yellow coating, and the pulse is wiry and rapid.

【Pathomechanism】

"Excessive qi can transform into fire". When patterns of liver qi stagnation associated with emotional changes are not treated correctly or promptly, the excessive qi can transform internally into fire. The liver regulates emotion and also connects with the orifice of the eyes, and a branch of the liver channel also connects to the vertex of the head. Internal fire will disturb the functions of the liver, causing stagnation that interrupts the smooth flow of qi.

Clinical manifestations of liver qi stagnation with liver fire include irritability and a burning pain in the hypochondriac region. Internal fire can also ascend the liver channel divergence to attack the head and the eyes, causing severe headache, red eyes, and reddish facial complexion. Ascending liver fire can also disturb the spirit to cause insomnia and nightmares.

The liver and gallbladder stand in an interior-exterior relationship, with a branch of the gallbladder channel connecting with the ears. Thus, internal fire can move from the liver channel to the gallbladder channel, resulting in tinnitus as well as an over-production of bile that will result in a bitter taste in the mouth.

Fire can also reduce body fluids to cause thirst with a propensity for cold drinks, dry stools, and dark yellow urine. The red tongue with a yellow coating and wiry rapid pulses are both indications of liver depression transforming into fire.

【Treatment Principle】

Clear liver fire, move liver qi.

【Prescription】

Modified *Dān Zhī Xiāo Yáo Sǎn* (Free Wanderer Powder plus Cortex Moutan and Fructus Gardeniae)

柴胡	*chái hú*	10g	Radix Bupleuri
白芍	*bái sháo*	15g	Radix Paeoniae Alba
丹皮	*dān pí*	10g	Cortex Moutan
栀子	*zhī zǐ*	10g	Fructus Gardeniae
当归	*dāng guī*	10g	Radix Angelicae Sinensis

continued

茯苓	*fú líng*	10g	Poria
白术	*bái zhú*	10g	Rhizoma Atractylodis Macrocephalae
生姜	*shēng jiāng*	10g	Rhizoma Zingiberis Recens
薄荷	*bò hé*	6g	Herba Menthae
甘草	*gān cǎo*	6g	Radix et Rhizoma Glycyrrhizae

【Formula Analysis】

Chái hú (Radix Bupleuri) acts to soothe the liver, relieve depression, and promote the free flow of liver qi, where *dāng guī* (Radix Angelicae Sinensis) and *bái sháo* (Radix Paeoniae Alba) nourish blood. Combined, these three medicinals act to regulate the liver while harmonizing and nourishing blood.

Because disease can easily transmute from liver-wood to spleen-earth, *fú líng* (Poria), *bái zhú* (Rhizoma Atractylodis Macrocephalae) and *gān cǎo* (Radix et Rhizoma Glycyrrhizae) are used to strengthen the spleen and replenish qi.

Dān pí (Cortex Moutan), *zhī zǐ* (Fructus Gardeniae), and *bò hé* (Herba Menthae) act to clear heat in the liver channel, and *shēng jiāng* (Rhizoma Zingiberis Recens) harmonizes the middle *jiao*.

【Modifications】

➢ With dry mouth, add *tiān huā fěn* (Radix Trichosanthis) 20g and *shí hú* (Caulis Dendrobii) 10g to promote fluid production and relieve thirst.

➢ With a bitter taste in the mouth, add *huáng qín* (Radix Scutellariae Hypericifoliae) 10g to clear liver fire and promote gallbladder function.

➢ With irritability, add *xià kū cǎo* (Spica Prunellae) 20g to soothe the liver and subdue yang.

➢ With vexation, add *huáng lián* (Rhizoma Coptidis) 10g and *dàn dòu chǐ* (Semen Sojae Praeparatum) 10g to clear heart heat and relieve vexation.

➢ With insomnia and nightmares, add *lóng gǔ* (Os Draconis) 20 to 30g to soothe the liver and calm the spirit.

➢ With dry stools, add *dà huáng* (Radix et Rhizoma Rhei) 3 to 6g to discharge large intestine heat.

➢ With severe headaches, add *gōu téng* (Ramulus Uncariae Cum Uncis) 30g (decocted later) and *chuān xiōng* (Rhizoma Chuanxiong) to soothe the liver and relieve pain.

(3) Exuberant Heart Fire

【Signs and Symptoms】

Hypervigilance, irritability, vexation, difficulty falling asleep, vexing heat in the chest, palms and soles, dizziness, tinnitus, lower back pain, seminal emission, a red complexion, mouth and tongue ulcers, dry mouth, delirious speech, mania, dry stools and painful urination with dark yellow urine. The tongue is red with a dry coating, and the pulse is rapid and thready.

【Pathomechanism】

Extended periods of anxiety give rise to qi stagnation, often resulting in the accumulation of internal heat which tends to rise upward to disquiet the heart. Heart fire disturbs the spirit, with clinical manifestations of vexation, insomnia, and mania. Fire also reduces body fluids resulting in thirst and constipation. Branches of the heart channel may become affected to manifest with vexation in the chest, a red complexion, tongue and mouth ulcers, and a red tongue.

The heart and small intestine stand in an interior-exterior relationship, so internal heat can transfer from the heart channel to the small intestine channel to cause difficult and painful urination with dark yellow urine. Heart fire can also lead to non-interaction of heart and kidney, which may also cause seminal emission.

【Treatment Principle】

Clear heat, calm the spirit.

【Prescription】

Modified *Dǎo Chì Sǎn* (Red Guiding Powder) and *Jiāo Tài Wán* (Coordinate Heart and Kidney Pills)

生地	*shēng dì*	20g	Radix Rehmanniae
川木通	*chuān mù tōng*	6g	Caulis Clematidis Armandii
淡竹叶	*dàn zhú yè*	15g	Herba Lophatheri
肉桂	*ròu guì*	6g	Cortex Cinnamomi

continued

黄连	*huáng lián*	6g	Rhizoma Coptidis
茯神	*fú shén*	30g	Sclerotium Poriae Pararadicis
夜交藤	*yè jiāo téng*	30g	Caulis Polygoni Multiflori
菊花	*jú huā*	15g	Flos Chrysanthemi
桑叶	*sāng yè*	10g	Folium Mori

【Formula Analysis】

Sweet and cool *shēng dì* (Radix Rehmanniae) acts to cool the blood and nourish yin, and bitter and cold *chuān mù tōng* (Caulis Clematidis Armandii) enters the heart and small intestine channels to clear heart fire and small intestine heat. Combined, these two medicinals act to nourish yin and promote urination without impairing yin.

Huáng lián (Rhizoma Coptidis) clears heart fire and relieves vexation by guiding fire to its origin; it also clears internal heat by promoting urination when combined with *ròu guì* (Cortex Cinnamomi).

Dàn zhú yè (Herba Lophatheri), *fú shén* (Sclerotium Poriae Pararadicis), and *yè jiāo téng* (Caulis Polygoni Multiflori) act to calm the spirit.

Jú huā (Flos Chrysanthemi) and *sāng yè* (Folium Mori) clear liver heat while also helping to clear heart fire.

【Modifications】

➢ With dark yellow urine, add *huá shí* (Talcum) 20g and *fú líng* (Poria) 20g to promote urination.

➢ With ulcers of the tongue and mouth, add *huái shān yào* (Rhizoma Dioscoreae) 20g and *qīng dài* (Indigo Naturalis) 6g to clear heat, strengthen the spleen, and heal sores.

➢ With tinnitus and deafness, add *chán tuì* (Periostracum Cicadae) 10g and *shí chāng pú* (Rhizoma Acori Tatarinowii) 10g to open the orifices.

➢ With spontaneous seminal emission, add baked *lóng gǔ* (Os Draconis) 20g and baked *mǔ lì* (Concha Ostreae).

➢ For uncontrollable twitching, add *gān cǎo* (Radix et Rhizoma Glycyrrhizae Praeparata cum Melle) 6g, *xiǎo mài* (Fructus Tritici) 30g and *dà zǎo* (Fructus Jujubae) 15g as contained in the formula

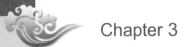

Gān Mài Dà Zǎo Tāng (Licorice, Wheat and Jujube Decoction) from *Essentials from the Golden Cabinet* (*Jīn Guì Yào Lüè*) to moisten sinews, strengthen the spleen, and nourish the heart.

(4) Phlegm-Fire Disturbing the Heart and Gallbladder
【Signs and Symptoms】

Hyperarousal, insomnia, recurring and disturbing dreams of the traumatic event, easily frightened, frequent nightmares, dizziness, stuffiness and fullness in the stomach and abdomen, a bitter taste in the mouth, vomiting and nausea, excessive and random speech, excessive exercising, aggression, poor appetite, and a sticky or greasy sensation in the mouth with abundant sputum. The tongue is red with a yellow greasy coating, and the pulse is wiry and slippery or rapid and slippery.

【Pathomechanism】

The liver and gallbladder stand in an interior-exterior relationship, and both organs are associated with emotion. The gallbladder governs decision, so normal gallbladder function promotes sound judgment and decisiveness. However, fright and emotional instability will lead to dysfunction of both liver and gallbladder.

Qi stagnation can cause the internal accumulation of phlegm; this can transform into fire which tends to rise, affecting the heart and disquieting the spirit. Phlegm-fire can affect both heart and gallbladder, resulting in clinical manifestations of vexation, insomnia, dreaminess, and palpitation. Phlegm-fire also leads to disharmony of the gallbladder and stomach with manifestations of dizziness and vomiting fluids.

Phlegm can affect the mind, resulting in clinical dizziness and even epilepsy. As phlegm-fire disturbs the heart-spirit, excessive ranting or aggressive behavior may appear. Phlegm obstruction and qi stagnation impairs splenic transformation and transportation, resulting in excessive sputum and poor appetite. A red tongue with a greasy yellow coating and wiry and slippery or rapid slippery pulses are also indications of phlegm-fire disturbing the heart and the gallbladder.

【Treatment Principle】

Clear heat, resolve phlegm, calm the spirit.

【Prescription】

Modified *Wēn Dǎn Tāng* (Gallbladder-Warming Decoction)

竹茹	*zhú rú*	10g	Caulis Bambusae in Taenia
枳实	*zhǐ shí*	12g	Fructus Aurantii Immaturus
陈皮	*chén pí*	15g	Pericarpium Citri Reticulatae
清半夏	*qīng bàn xià*	10g	Rhizoma Pinelliae Concisum
茯苓	*fú líng*	20g	Poria
生姜	*shēng jiāng*	10g	Rhizoma Zingiberis Recens
白术	*bái zhú*	10g	Rhizoma Atractylodis Macrocephalae
大枣	*dà zǎo*	12g	Fructus Jujubae
槟榔	*bīng láng*	10g	Semen Arecae
甘草	*gān cǎo*	6g	Radix et Rhizoma Glycyrrhizae Praeparata cum Melle

【Formula Analysis】

Pungent and warm *bàn xià* (Rhizoma Pinelliae) acts to dry dampness, resolve phlegm, harmonize the stomach and stop vomiting, while sweet and cold *zhú rú* (Caulis Bambusae in Taenia) clears heat, resolves phlegm, relieves vexation, and stops vomiting.

Pungent and bitter and warm *chén pí* (Pericarpium Citri Reticulatae) regulates qi, dries dampness, and resolves phlegm, while *zhǐ shí* (Fructus Aurantii Immaturus) and *bīng láng* (Semen Arecae) downbear qi, remove food stagnation, resolve phlegm, and dissolve masses.

Fú líng (Poria) strengthens the spleen and eliminates dampness; *shēng jiāng* (Rhizoma Zingiberis Recens) and *dà zǎo* (Fructus Jujubae) harmonize spleen and stomach, and *shēng jiāng* (Rhizoma Zingiberis Recens) reduces the toxicity of *bàn xià* (Rhizoma Pinelliae).

Generally speaking, *chén pí* (Pericarpium Citri Reticulatae), *bàn xià* (Rhizoma Pinelliae), and *shēng jiāng* (Rhizoma Zingiberis Recens) display warming properties, while *zhú rú* (Caulis Bambusae in Taenia) and *zhǐ shí* (Fructus Aurantii Immaturus) are cooling. These medicinals in combination form a balanced formula that acts to regulate qi, harmonize the stomach, and resolve phlegm to effectively restore gallbladder function.

【Modifications】

➢ With frequent nightmares, add *lóng gǔ* (Os Draconis) 20g, *mǔ lì* (Concha Ostreae) and *zhēn zhū mǔ* (Concha Margaritiferae Usta)

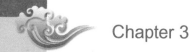

20g to tranquilize the spirit.

> With unconsciousness, add *shí chāng pú* (Rhizoma Acori Tatarinowii) 10g and *yuǎn zhì* (Radix Polygalae) 10g to resolve phlegm and open the orifices.

> With white-colored phlegm, add *bái jiè zǐ* (Semen Sinapis) 15g and *zǐ sū zǐ* (Fructus Perillae) 10g to resolve phlegm and dissipate masses.

> With yellow sticky phlegm, add *zhì nán xīng* (Arisaema cum Bile) 6g and *zhì yuǎn zhì* (Radix Polygalae) 6g to clear heat, and resolve phlegm.

> With poor appetite, add *shén qū* (Massa Medicata Fermentata) 15g and *shān zhā* (Fructus Crataegi) 15g to strengthen the spleen and harmonize the stomach.

> With abdominal distention, add *mù xiāng* (Radix Aucklandiae) 15g and *hòu pò* (Cortex Magnoliae Officinalis) 10g to regulate qi and eliminate food stagnation.

DEFICIENCY PATTERNS

(1) Deficiency of Heart and Spleen
【Signs and Symptoms】

Hypervigilance, emotional disturbance, dizziness, mental fatigue, palpitation, timidity, insomnia, poor memory, poor appetite, pale lips and a pale complexion. The tongue is pale with thin white coating, and the pulse is thready and weak.

【Pathomechanism】

Internal damage from the seven emotions (i.e. excessive over-thinking) can lead to the consumption of blood and poor nourishment of the spleen and heart that causes disquieting of the spirit. The heart controls the spirit and governs the vessels, and the spleen governs thinking and controls blood. Over-thinking results in consumption of spleen qi and heart blood.

Spleen qi deficiency manifests with fatigue and a poor appetite, and heart blood deficiency causes malnourishment of the heart that leads to emotional disorders, fright palpitations, severe anxiety, poor memory, and insomnia. The pale complexion, pale tongue, and weak thready pulses are all indications of spleen qi deficiency and heart blood deficiency.

【Treatment Principle】

Nourish heart blood, tonify spleen qi.

【Prescription】

Modified *Guī Pí Tāng* (Spleen-Restoring Decoction)

人参	*rén shēn*	15g	Radix et Rhizoma Ginseng
白术	*bái zhú*	15g	Rhizoma Atractylodis Macrocephalae
茯苓	*fú líng*	15g	Poria
炙黄芪	*zhì huáng qí*	10g	Radix Astragali Praeparata cum Melle
龙眼肉	*lóng yǎn ròu*	15g	Arillus Longan
酸枣仁	*suān zǎo rén*	15g	Semen Ziziphi Spinosae
木香	*mù xiāng*	9g	Radix Aucklandiae
当归	*dāng guī*	10g	Radix Angelicae Sinensis
远志	*yuǎn zhì*	10g	Radix Polygalae
大枣	*dà zǎo*	12g	Fructus Jujubae
生姜	*shēng jiāng*	10g	Rhizoma Zingiberis Recens
甘草	*gān cǎo*	9g	Radix et Rhizoma Glycyrrhizae

【Formula Analysis】

The formula mainly focuses on tonification of the spleen, since the spleen is the source of qi and blood. In this formula, sweet and warm *rén shēn* (Radix et Rhizoma Ginseng), *bái zhú* (Rhizoma Atractylodis Macrocephalae), *fú líng* (Poria) and *gān cǎo* (Radix et Rhizoma Glycyrrhizae) all act to tonify the spleen to promote the production of blood.

Sweet and warm *dāng guī* (Radix Angelicae Sinensis) and *lóng yǎn ròu* (Arillus Longan) act to tonify heart blood, while *suān zǎo rén* (Semen Ziziphi Spinosae), *yuǎn zhì* (Radix Polygalae) and *fú líng* (Poria) calm the spirit.

Pungent *mù xiāng* (Radix Aucklandiae) regulates qi and strengthens the spleen, also acting in concert with the other tonifying medicinals in the formula to help the spleen regain its function of transformation.

Dà zǎo (Fructus Jujubae) and *shēng jiāng* (Rhizoma Zingiberis Recens) act to harmonize the spleen and stomach.

【Modifications】

➢ With vertigo, add *chuān xiōng* (Rhizoma Chuanxiong) 10g and *gǒu qǐ zǐ* (Fructus Lycii) 15g to tonify the kidney and activate blood.

➢ With palpitation and timidity, add *hǔ pò* (Succinum) 15g and *zhēn zhū mǔ* (Concha Margaritiferae Usta) 20g to tranquilize the spirit.

➢ With poor memory, add *shú dì huáng* (Radix Rehmanniae Praeparata) 20g to tonify kidney yin.

➢ With insomnia and nightmares, add *bǎi hé* (Bulbus Lilii) 30g and *bǎi zǐ rén* (Semen Platycladi) to nourish the heart and calm the spirit.

(2) Qi Deficiency of Heart and Gallbladder
【Signs and Symptoms】

Palpitations, timidity, difficulty falling asleep, frequent nightmares, fear of experiencing a similar traumatic event, dizziness, blurred vision, shortness of breath and fatigue. The tongue is pale tongue with white coating, and the pulse is wiry and thready.

【Pathomechanism】

Fright leads to qi dysfunction and the heart fails to govern the spirit resulting in palpitations, poor sleep quality, nightmares, dizziness and blurred vision. Gallbladder qi deficiency can affect the stomach resulting in vomiting and nausea and shortness of breath. The pale tongue and wiry and thready pulses are both indications of qi deficiency of the heart and gallbladder.

【Treatment Principle】

Tranquilize the mind, calm the spirit.

【Prescription】

Modified *Ān Shén Dìng Zhì Wán* (Tranquilizing Mind Pills)

人参	*rén shēn*	10g	Radix et Rhizoma Ginseng
茯苓	*fú líng*	20g	Poria
柏子仁	*bǎi zǐ rén*	15g	Semen Platycladi
酸枣仁	*suān zǎo rén*	15g	Semen Ziziphi Spinosae
石菖蒲	*shí chāng pú*	10g	Rhizoma Acori Tatarinowii
当归	*dāng guī*	10g	Radix Angelicae Sinensis

continued

远志	*yuǎn zhì*	10g	Radix Polygalae
琥珀	*hǔ pò*	20g	Succinum (wrap-boiled)

【**Formula Analysis**】

Rén shēn (Radix et Rhizoma Ginseng) acts to tonify qi and *dāng guī* (Radix Angelicae Sinensis) nourishes blood, together they nourish both heart and gallbladder.

Yuǎn zhì (Radix Polygalae), *fú líng* (Poria), and *shí chāng pú* (Rhizoma Acori Tatarinowii) resolve phlegm, eliminate dampness, and open the orifices.

Hǔ pò (Succinum) tranquilizes the mind, while *bǎi zǐ rén* (Semen Platycladi) and *suān zǎo rén* (Semen Ziziphi Spinosae) nourish the heart and calm the spirit.

【**Modifications**】

➢ With insomnia and fluid damage due to sweating, add *Suān Zǎo Rén Tāng* (Sour Jujube Decoction) to astringe fluids while calming the mind and spirit.

➢ With shortness of breath and fatigue, add *huáng qí* (Radix Astragali) 20g, *bái zhú* (Rhizoma Atractylodis Macrocephalae), and *huái shān yào* (Rhizoma Dioscoreae) to strengthen the spleen and tonify qi.

➢ With palpitation and fear, add *lóng gǔ* (Os Draconis, baked) and *mǔ lì* (Concha Ostreae, baked) to calm the spirit.

(3) Non-interaction of Heart and Kidney

【**Signs and Symptoms**】

Hyperarousal, difficulty falling asleep, frequent nightmares, vexation, dizziness, tinnitus, tidal fever, night sweats, seminal emission and impotence, menstrual disorders, poor memory, palpitations, tongue and mouth ulcers, and dry stools. The tongue is red with little coating, and the pulse is rapid and thready.

【**Pathomechanism**】

Excessive mental activity leads to a disharmony of heart fire and kidney water with non-interaction of heart and kidney, and yin deficiency of the heart and kidney leads to effulgent hyperactive fire. Fire tends to rise upward to disturb the spirit, manifesting with vexation, insomnia, palpitations and dream-disturbed sleep.

Deficiency of kidney yin, bone marrow deficiency, and poor nourishment of the brain manifests with dizziness, tinnitus, poor memory, and soreness of the lower back and knees.

Effulgent internal fire affects the kidney to cause seminal emission and impotence, vexing heat in the chest, palms and soles, tidal fever, night sweats, and tongue and mouth ulcers. The red tongue with a scanty coating and rapid thready pulses are all indications of heart and kidney non-interaction.

【Treatment Principle】

Tonify yin, nourish blood, calm the spirit, harmonize heart and kidney.

【Prescription】

Modified *Tiān Wáng Bǔ Xīn Dān* (Celestial Emperor Heart-Supplementing Elixir)

生地	*shēng dì*	30g	Radix Rehmanniae
玄参	*xuán shēn*	15g	Radix Scrophulariae
天冬	*tiān dōng*	15g	Radix Asparagi
麦冬	*mài dōng*	20g	Radix Ophiopogonis
丹参	*dān shēn*	15g	Radix et Rhizoma Salviae Miltiorrhizae
人参	*rén shēn*	10g	Radix et Rhizoma Ginseng
酸枣仁	*suān zǎo rén*	20g	Semen Ziziphi Spinosae
当归	*dāng guī*	10g	Radix Angelicae Sinensis
五味子	*wǔ wèi zǐ*	12g	Fructus Schisandrae Chinensis
桔梗	*jié gěng*	10g	Radix Platycodonis
柏子仁	*bǎi zǐ rén*	15g	Semen Platycladi
黄连	*huáng lián*	10g	Rhizoma Coptidis
肉桂	*ròu guì*	5g	Cortex Cinnamomi
茯苓	*fú líng*	20g	Poria
远志	*yuǎn zhì*	10g	Radix Polygalae

【Formula Analysis】

Sweet and cold *shēng dì* (Radix Rehmanniae) acts to nourish heart blood and tonify kidney yin, and *dāng guī* (Radix Angelicae Sinensis) tonifies blood and nourishes yin.

Tiān dōng (Radix Asparagi) and *mài dōng* (Radix Ophiopogonis) tonifies the kidney and clears heat, and *xuán shēn* (Radix Scrophulariae) nourishes yin and clears heat.

Suān zǎo rén (Semen Ziziphi Spinosae), *bǎi zǐ rén* (Semen Platycladi), *fú líng* (Poria) and *yuǎn zhì* (Radix Polygalae) all act to nourish the heart and calm the spirit.

Wǔ wèi zǐ (Fructus Schisandrae Chinensis) astringes heart qi and calms the spirit, while *rén shēn* (Radix et Rhizoma Ginseng) acts to tonify qi, calm the spirit, and improve memory.

Dān shēn (Radix et Rhizoma Salviae Miltiorrhizae) clears heart fire and actives blood, while *huáng lián* (Rhizoma Coptidis) and *ròu guì* (Cortex Cinnamomi) clear heart fire and guide fire back to its origin. Also as a guiding herb, *jié gěng* (Radix Platycodonis) acts to guide the medicinal action towards the heart.

This formula combination aims to improve heart and kidney function by nourishing blood and yin (anchoring the root) and calming the spirit (treating the branch).

【Modifications】

➤ With tongue and mouth ulcers, add *chuān mù tōng* (Caulis Clematidis Armandii) 10g, and *dàn zhú yè* (Herba Lophatheri) 10g to clear heart and promote urination.

➤ With tidal fever and night sweating, add *fú xiǎo mài* (Fructus Tritici Levis) 30g to astringe sweat.

➤ With dry stools, add *ròu cōng róng* (Herba Cistanches) 20g to nourish yin and relax the bowels.

Tui-na Acupressure Self-massage

In addition to receiving massage therapy in the clinic, PTSD patients may also benefit from self-massage applied to the following acupressure points.

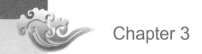
(1) Point *tài yáng* **(EX-HN5)**

Location: On the temples, in the depression one finger-width posterior to the midpoint of the line linking the end of the eyebrow and outer canthus of the eye.

Manipulation: Use a kneading movement with the index and middle fingers moving clockwise for eight-beats, and then counter-clockwise. Repeat as needed.

(2) Point *yìn táng* **(EX-HN3)**

Location: On the forehead, midway between the medial ends of the two eyebrows.

Manipulation: Use a scrubbing movement with the thumb, scrubbing upward from the bridge of the nose to the anterior hairline for eight beats. Pause and repeat.

(3) GB 20 (*fēng chí***)**

Location: On the posterior aspect of the neck at the base of the skull, in the depression between the upper portion of the sternocleidomastoid and trapezius muscles.

Manipulation: Use a kneading movement with the index, middle, and ring fingers moving clockwise for eight-beats, and then counter-clockwise. Repeat as needed.

(4) PC 8 (*láo gōng***)**

Location: On the transverse crease of the palm, between the 2nd and 3rd metacarpal bones.

Manipulation: Use a kneading movement with the thumb moving clockwise for eight-beats, and then counter-clockwise. Repeat as needed.

(5) PC 6 (*nèi guān***)**

Location: 2 *cun* above the transverse crease of the inner wrist, between the two tendons of m. palmaris longus and m. flexor carpi radialis.

Manipulation: Press the point heavily with the thumb, and pause. Repeat for 8 beats, continue as needed.

(6) SJ 5 (*wài guān***)**

Location: 2 *cun* above the transverse crease of the outer aspect of the wrist, between the radius and ulna.

Manipulation: Press the point heavily with the thumb, and pause. Repeat for 8 beats, continue as needed.

(7) HT 7 (*shén mén*)

Location: On the ulnar end of transverse crease of the wrist, in the depression on the radial side of the tendon of m. flexor carpi ulnaris.

Manipulation: Press the point heavily with the thumb, and pause. Repeat for 8 beats, continue as needed.

(8) Auricular Massage

Location: The external ear and ear lobes.

Manipulation: With thumb and index finger holding the ear, rub the auricle from top to bottom, and from inside to outside. Repeat for 8 beats, continue as needed.

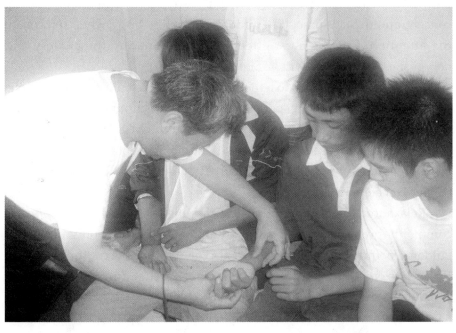

Teaching *tui-na* self-massage

Qi-gong Therapy

Qi-gong therapy generally includes conduction exercises, breathwork,

Chapter 3

and meditation techniques. Such exercise aims to control and regulate the qi dynamic, as reflected by the term *"qi gong"* (qi cultivation). Many of these exercises were first innovated during the Spring and Autumn and Warring States Periods, although further development has continued throughout history. Hua Tuo's "five animal exercises" and Zhang San-feng's tai-chi boxing exercises both contain Qi-gong principles within them.

Qi-gong therapy should be practiced only with an experienced practitioner because some exercises have been known to cause a state of psychosis when performed incorrectly. Initial symptoms may include numbness of the extremities, agitation, hypertension, depression, insomnia, anxiety, nausea, vertigo, soreness and pain, and dizziness.

Qi-gong can be categorized into internal, external, dynamic, static, martial, life-cultivating and disease-treating exercises. All of them focus on three aspects, namely "body regulation" (generalized relaxation, also known as postures), "breath regulation" and "spirit regulation" (mental concentration). Such practices gradually relax the body while refocusing the attention, and are most effective for eliminating the anxiety and nervousness associated with PTSD.

Spirit regulation refers to a method that involves both relaxation of the body while focusing upon specific body parts or acupuncture points with the intention of eliminating miscellaneous thoughts. Generally, mental concentration is focused on or below the umbilicus. Body regulation and breath regulation methods are actually rooted in regulation of the spirit, so they can be practiced together.

Relaxation exercises, emotional release methods, and *Ba Duan Jin* are commonly prescribed, but again, patients must practice only under the guidance of qualified therapists, and also understand the contraindications for each exercise. If any physical discomfort occurs during practice, one should seek medical care immediately.

Also be sure to adhere to the following practice guidelines:

1. Within a half an hour before practice, stop all heavy physical activities and settle the mood. Also remove all accessories such as hats, glasses, watches and bracelets. The practitioner should not be excessively hungry or full, and the body should be kept warm. Drinking a small amount of warm water can promote the

movement of qi and blood, and warm-up exercises that relax the muscles and joints can also be conducted at this time.

2. After practice, bathing or hand washing with cold water is prohibited. Drinking cold beverages immediately after practice is also prohibited. With sweating, wipe down with a dry towel or wash with hot water.

QI-GONG METHODS

Relaxation Exercises
Basic Principles

1) The following relaxation and breathing exercises can be done either standing, sitting or lying down; weak people with chronic physical conditions may practice while lying down. With standing or sitting practices, one can slightly open the eyes; if there is difficulty in standing in a stable position, the eyes should remain open.

2) At the beginning of practice, the breath is natural; the practice abdominal breathing may be entered into gradually.

3) The mind should focus on the relaxed feelings of the muscles, also using one's intention to induce further relaxation. Over time this practice becomes an unconscious effort.

Methods
1) Relaxation according to parts

Mentally divide the body into several horizontal parts and relax sequentially from the top to the bottom. For example, first relax the head to shoulders, then the shoulders to hips (the upper limbs should also relax from shoulders to hands), and at lastly from the hips to feet. This is called "three-part relaxation" , and breathing exercises are often employed at the same time. When practicing while sitting down, relaxing the body parts above the hip is sufficient.

2) Relaxation according to lines

Visualize virtual lines on the body and relax them accordingly. For example, imagine the first line going from the head along the spine to the sacrum; the second line runs from the shoulders to the hands; and the third line goes from the hips to the feet. This can be referred to as "three-line

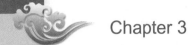

relaxation". When practicing, also pay attention to the breath.

3) Breathwork

Regulation of the breath is based on natural breathing, where over time the breath becomes fine, even, deep, and long. Similar to yogic breathwork, there are also techniques for abdominal breathing, anus-lifting breathing, and rapid breathing, all of which can be combined with the intoning or sub-vocalization of selected syllables or words. Each variation can be applied for different conditions in accordance with pattern differentiation. For example, anus-lifting breathing is recommended for patients with spleen qi fall, and rapid breathing is appropriate for those with heart blood insufficiency or vexation and agitation.

The following exercise primarily aims to instruct the patient in the method of abdominal breathing so that the patient can learn to regulate their emotions independently. It is useful for not only relieving the emotional pain caused by the trauma, but it can also strengthen mental function.

a. The patient sits on a chair with the bottoms of both feet touching the ground. Leaning against the back of the chair, relax the shoulders and legs with hands placed on both knees.

b. The therapist sits on a chair of the same height, to the right of the patient. His knees should be positioned at a 45–60 degree angle to the patient's legs.

c. Perform abdominal deep breathing in a long and slow manner. When inhaling, focus on the lower abdomen, feeling the expansion of the abdomen and lumbar region. With even deeper inhalations, feel that the legs and feet are expanding as well, with the body connected to the earth through the feet. When exhaling, focus the mind upon the shoulders with the neck and shoulders expanding and relaxing. With even deeper exhalation, feel the sensation of relaxation as extending to the back, lumbus, and legs, with the body connected to the earth through the feet.

Notes:

◆ The physician should conduct every step of the exercise with a calm and deeply suggestive tone of voice as well as with suggestive choice of words.

◆ When the patient is experiencing mood swings or having difficulties relaxing, the physician may place his left palm onto the sixth and seventh cervical vertebra of the patient, with the index finger and thumb of his right hand on the patient's forehead.

4) Mind-Spirit Quieting Therapy

This therapy helps patients to acquire a status of "not being disturbed by troublesome thoughts from the inside, and not being taxed by things in the outside world" . Such methods include sitting, lying or standing meditation techniques and other methods of self-discipline. Clinically, meditation acts to strengthen the upright qi in order to help prevent or eliminate disease. When using this therapy, one should also pay attention to the weather and climate of the four seasons, and focus the mind accordingly; for example, an unconstrained mood may be cultivated in the springtime because everything in nature is growing. This idea reflects the Chinese naturalistic viewpoint of "heaven and humankind are mutually responsive" .

5) Subvocalization

The subvocalization or intoning of specific syllables or positive words can help eliminate troublesome thoughts so that one can relax, similar the yoga practice of mantra repetition. This technique provides an optimum stimulation to the cerebral cortex, which takes effect through the secondary signal system. The choice of words or syllables may vary according to the patient's condition. For example, patients with high blood pressure or neurosis with predominant excitement tend to be anxious and nervous. In this case, words like "relax" and "quiet" can be combined with the breath, one for inhalation and the other for exhalation. Meanwhile, conduct the intention to relax downwards. Others may select syllables that correspond with the internal organs as described in Taoist alchemical practices, or mantras that correspond with the chakra system as described in yoga.

Emotional Release

This exercise from the *Mǎ Wáng Duī Yī Shū: Dǎo Yǐn Tú* (*Medical Book

from Ma Wang Dui: Illustrations of Conduction Exercises) involves breathing, movement, and focused intention. This particular technique is most effective for treating disorders of the qi dynamic caused by anger and anxiety.

For the preparatory posture, stand erect with the feet shoulder-width apart with both arms extended forward, palms facing forward. The body should be entirely relaxed with the lower lip protruding slightly forward. Relax and breathe naturally, moving the hands toward the body while inhaling deeply from the chest to the lower abdomen. Hold for one second.

While exhaling slowly, the breath moves upwards through the chest, diaphragm, and mouth while making a slight hissing sound. At the same time, slowly straighten the elbows, pushing the palms forward to reach their original position. Exhale fully until there is a slightly suffocating sensation. The intention here is to slowly release any accumulated anger, hatred, oppression, and internal fullness along with the out-breath. Stand still for a short while and repeat the same sequence of movement for eleven more repetitions.

Ba Duan Jin

Ba Duan Jin exercises date back to the Song Dynasty, and it remains one of the most commonly used Qi-gong forms. More commonly known as Eight Pieces of Brocade or the Eight Silken Movements, the name of the form generally refers to how the eight individual movements of the form are characterized by a silken quality (like a piece of brocade). The *Ba Duan Jin* form is broken down into eight sections, each of which focuses on a different area of the body. The routine enhances limb strength and flexibility of the joints, and benefits the nerves. Often used in the treatment osteoporosis, it has also been shown to improve the respiratory, cardiovascular and immune systems. Like all self-cultivation methods, it can also benefit one's mental health.

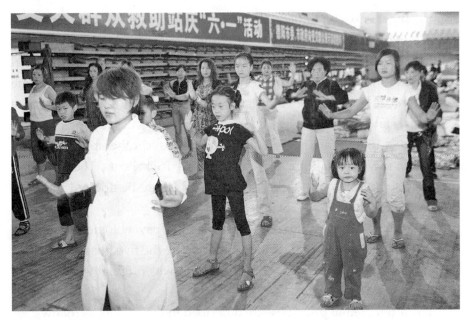

Group *qi-gong* practice in Sichuan

Tai-chi

When practicing tai-chi or tai-chi sword forms, the muscles of the whole body should remain relaxed with gentle movements that promote a feeling of ease. Relaxed muscles and nerves can lower blood pressure, and the movements of the muscles and joints improve motor function. During practice, the breathing is deep, long and even, and movements of the hip are emphasized. These techniques improve blood circulation in the abdominal cavity, eliminate blood stasis, promote bowel movements, and can attenuate pathological changes of the digestive tract. Therefore, tai-chi exercise benefits PTSD patients by not only helping relieve their anxiety, but also by creating balance among the internal organs while also promoting recovery from physical damage. The twenty-four movement tai-chi form and the thirty-two movement tai-chi sword forms are most commonly used.

TCM Psychotherapy

In Chinese medicine, the human emotions are summarized by the seven affects as described in Chapter 2, and also the "five minds" which

are joy, anger, anxiety, thought and fear. The seven affects and five minds characterize our subjective experience towards external stimulation, and yet they are also the manifestations of organ function. Different emotional stimuli affect each organ differently. Any emotion in excess can become a primary cause of disease, but the proper facilitation of an appropriate emotional state can also act as a cure.

Editor's note: Practitioners unlicensed in psychotherapy should not attempt to perform "talk therapy" with their PTSD clients. The following methods should be considered carefully, and only be applied by those qualified within their scope of practice.

Emotional-restraint therapy is a fast-acting psychological technique that employs the restraining relationships among the five phases as related to the five minds. This approach to treatment was originally recorded in the *The Yellow Emperor's Inner Classic*.

The fundamental principles are described in the classics as follows:

➢ Wood restrains earth. Excessive thought damages spleen-earth, which is restrained by liver-wood. Resolve this with anger.

➢ Earth restrains water. Extreme fear damages kidney-water, which is restrained by spleen-earth. Resolve this with thought.

➢ Water restrains fire. Excessive joy damages heart-fire, which is restrained by kidney-water. Resolve this with fear.

➢ Fire restrains metal. Extreme anxiety damages lung-metal, which is restrained by heart-fire. Resolve this with joy.

➢ Metal restrains wood. Excessive anger damages liver-wood, which is restrained by lung-metal. Resolve this with anxiety.

The engendering and restraining relationships of the five phases can serve as a guide to treatment, but their applications in practice should remain flexible because the emotional activities of human beings are inherently complex. In any event, the root cause must be differentiated precisely before applying treatment of any kind.

Another classical approach to understanding the prevailing relationships between two emotions involves regulation of a third emotion:

➢ Anxiety prevails over anger, with regulation of fear.

➢ Fear prevails over joy, with regulation of anger.

➢ Joy prevails over anxiety, with regulation of thought.

➢ Thought prevails over fear, with regulation of anxiety.

➢ Anger prevails over thought, with regulation of joy.

Thought—According to *The Yellow Emperor's Inner Classic*, thought prevails over fear. For patients with fearful emotions, the therapist should apply reason and give guidance based on the cause of their fears. This approach can provide the patient with positive insights that can help them gradually release their fright and fear.

Sorrow—According to *The Yellow Emperor's Inner Classic*, sorrow prevails over anger. For patients with excessive anger, vexation, agitation, irascibility, or even the tendency to hit people or smash things, the therapist may attempt to suppress their pathological anger with ideas that induce sorrow.

Joy—According to *The Yellow Emperor's Inner Classic*, joy prevails over sorrow and anxiety. There are many ways to induce joy and laughter with humor and comedy. The key here is to build a good relationship with the patient and to create a relaxing and joyful therapeutic environment. This treatment method is very broadly and commonly applied.

Anger—According to *The Yellow Emperor's Inner Classic*, anger prevails over thought. This method is indicated for persistent anxiety and rumination, or for qi binding with extremely low spirits when the use of joy is ineffective. However, one should clearly understand the principle of "prevailing over it with anger, but resolving it with joy" . For those with excess patterns such as liver yang hyperactivity, liver fire ascending and heart fire exuberance, this method is absolutely prohibited. Provocative language or behavior may not be appropriate in many cases, especially when treating those with PTSD.

Fear—"Fear is the mind of the kidney-water, thus it prevails over the joy of heart-fire." According to *The Yellow Emperor's Inner Classic*, fear prevails over joy. Certain words or behavior can induce fear, thus suppressing uncontrollable and excessive joy as it manifests.

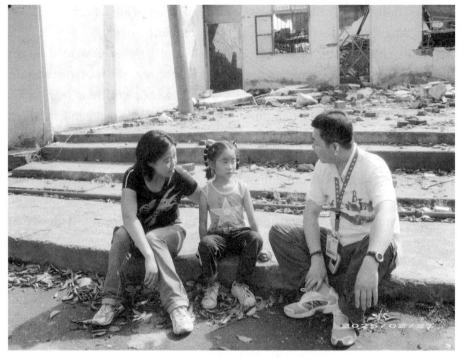

Counseling young earthquake survivors

FIVE-PHASE DIAGNOSIS

The Wood-type

When considering the wood-type, one first thinks of the obvious correspondences of springtime, wind, eyes, tears, shouting, anger, sour flavors, etc. However, there are other subtle features pertaining to this phase that are less obvious; these particular qualities can be of great value when determining a person's elemental or five-phase predominance.

For example, a wood-type PTSD patient will generally report anxiety, restless, and difficulty resting. The wood personality can be arrogant, confident, aggressive, confrontational, driven, and eager, often described as an "in your face" type of person. In wood cases, the primary issues involve control. They are very demanding of themselves as well because when they do not reach their goals, they feel a loss of control at which point they may fall into the clutches of depression. Usually, this type of depression involves a great well of repressed anger and disappointment with frustration brewing underneath the surface.

Regarding appearance, the wood-type presents with a reddish

complexion and eyes and a disgruntled countenance.

The Fire-type

The fire-type, on the other hand, has distinctly different features from those of the wood-type. The fire-type PTSD symptoms often will revolve around relationship problems. Fire-types display their moods on their sleeves, often with dependency issues affecting their relationships. Their depression is usually of a cyclical nature in that they tend to recover from heartbreak and then immediately move on to the next relationship.

Fire predominance leads to symptoms of anxiety, chest pain, frequent nightmares, a lack of joy, and depression. Depressive episodes readily deplete heart qi to cause the usual fire-related symptoms of palpitation, anxiety, shortness of breath, listlessness, and mental confusion (due to the heart's relationship to *shen*, or cognitive functioning). Fire-types exhibit an energetic vigor, but when depressed, they are often indifferent and listless. Because the heart governs blood, when the individual succumbs to stress and relational pressures, fire predominance lends itself to a host of blood-related mental problems.

Regarding appearance, fire-types tend to a reddish face with a rather pointy chin. Their hair tends to be curly, and when in balance they tend to move quickly and often appear to be in a rush.

The Earth-type

The earth-type often presents with the typically characteristic signs of digestive imbalance. Earth-types tend to over-eat during periods of depression and stress; they seek food for warmth and comfort. There is an energetic quality of centeredness, being grounded, peace, calm and compassion, but during bouts with depression, earth-types will display characteristics of dampness in that they become listless, emotionally heavy, and unmotivated. They can also shift into obsessive worry and over-concern.

The earth-type physical characteristics are unique, and usually quite obvious. Physically, earth-types are usually stocky and portly with rounded faces. They often fluctuate in weight during duress and depression, at yet, when they are balanced and healthy, earth-types exhibit a rather jovial appearance.

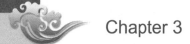

The Metal-type

Metal-type PTSD patients are extremely sensitive in regards to their surrounding environment. This type becomes depressed when loss and grief appears in their lives or work environment. Such emotions consume their vitality, and when unhealthy, this element characteristically presents with signs of upper respiratory infection or asthma.

When depressed, the metal type often sighs, cries, or sobs, often taking the sufferings of the world upon their shoulders. Therefore, this type may also involve a sense of grieving that seems to be overwhelming and all-encompassing. Metal-types are very sensitive to their surroundings and can even take on the emotions of others in a normal therapeutic setting.

Physically, metal-types have pale complexions, a weak appearance, and soft voices. When depressed, they appear very weak and meager. In many cases, these patients will have rather clear regrets, always wishing that things could have gone differently in the past. These people often feel plagued by circumstance, and therefore constantly grieve over their past issues and losses.

The Water-type

Water-types characteristically are the most dangerous types in the clinical setting and they are also the most difficult to treat. Often, their depressions are a result of genetics (pre-natal *jing*). The etiology of this type of depression is hard to comprehend; there is no insight as to what causes this five-phase type of depression.

These patients will display the most challenging psychological signs of schizophrenia, psychosis, and severe major depressive episodes. Typically, these patients become despondent, vegetative, and cannot perform normal activities. Their depression seems to show a darkness that eats away at their souls, becoming non-responsive and out of touch with their current reality. They are tormented with fears of life and death, and yet, they have no sense of what their fear means. They seem to have lost their sense of purpose in life are may even be reluctant to leave their homes; when they do leave their homes, someone usually accompanies them. They are often poorly groomed, scattered, fearful or apathetic, and they may also display nervous tremors. Water-types feel that they are beyond help, and they no longer seek assistance. Since they feel so lost, and because they cannot grasp what is plaguing them on such a pervasive and personal level, they often resort to suicide. These patients are most difficult types to treat successfully.

Summary

In each of the five-phase types discussed above, there are simple clues as to which phase is predominant. However, it is imperative to ask further questions to evoke the necessary information for a correct diagnosis. The use of the five-phase diagnosis is only one tool for dealing with post-traumatic stress disorder patients, but it does afford the practitioner an added sense of comprehension and clarity. However, it is also important to maintain focus on the most comprehensive and effective means of treatment. Comprehensive treatment needs to encompass an integrative approach involving psychotherapy as well as CAM modalities.

As alternative healthcare practitioners, it is also crucial to recognize the importance of dealing with the patient on a psychologically therapeutic level. In most cases of PTSD, there are unseen and underlying triggers that we as acupuncturists are not trained to deal with. The diagnostic process always keeps the best interests of the patient foremost in mind, and this requires both sensitivity and flexibility.

Although the theoretical model of the five phases can be useful in diagnosing and treating a patient suffering from PTSD, it is in fact only one diagnostic perspective. As stated previously, to assess the severity of the condition, a variety of diagnostic methods should be considered. In order to truly tend to the individual needs of each patient, PTSD must be dealt with on many levels.

TCM and Behavioral Therapy

Behavioral therapy in Chinese medicine follows the principles of pattern differentiation and also the restraining relationship among the five phases as described above. However, as compared to the pure TCM psychology approach, behavioral therapy displays some unique characteristics.

This type of therapy only aims at the present issue at hand, where the history of the issue or the visitor's self-knowledge and comprehension are

usually considered as irrelevant. Therapy focuses on the specific behaviors manifesting in the present moment. Behaviors that require change are usually considered as manifestations of psychological symptoms, so these techniques are based on behavioral practice.

Even though therapy can be carried out in the clinic, it is more significant that most of these techniques can be practiced by the client in daily life once he has learned the procedure. This approach also improves the patients' ability to adjust to different environments.

In a word, applied behavioral therapy does not include consideration of the subconscious mind or the essential causes of the internal mental status, nor the trends and consequence of the disease process. Instead, we focus on present and observable non-adaptive behavior. The main idea is that if the "behavior" changes, then the "attitude" and "emotion" will change accordingly. Additionally, behavioral therapy is more concerned about setting up a specific goal for treatment rather than the treatment procedure itself, with a specific goal set up after the physician observes the patient's behavior and functioning. Once the goal is clarified, a new learning process based on positive conditioning can begin.

In addition to the goal-setting discussed above, behavioral therapies include a wide variety of therapeutic techniques, but in this section we will only introduce those approaches deemed most appropriate for PTSD patients.

Adaptation

To PTSD patients, adaptation therapy mainly aims to diminish the information that triggers traumatic pain. This type of information includes images, hallucinations, thoughts, emotions and some biological activities of the body. Normally, this information is intrusive, re-experienced and negative. The therapy can only be carried out after the patient has performed relaxation exercises and both the physician and patient feel prepared. Contemporary "eye movement desensitization" is often combined here as well. The procedure is as follows:

After relaxation, both physician and patient keep the same sitting positions, and tell each other when they feel ready. First, the physician requires the patient to create a piece of negative "trigger information" in his mind that is related to the trauma. Then, characterize this "trigger information". For example, mentally highlight the intrusive image, hallucination or scene; the more pain it causes, the brighter it appears. Suggest that the resulting emotion can be gray or black; the more negative and painful the emotion is, the deeper the color. Do not trigger more than one piece of negative information at a time, especially during the initial course of treatment. Continue by telling the patient that during the next period of treatment, the brightness of the intrusive image will become reduced; the painful emotion will appear lighter in color; and the client's confidence in the treatment will increase. After inducing the "trigger information", related emotional pains and obstacles can become aggravated. Relaxation exercises should be repeated, usually through guided breathwork.

The next phase involves the therapist moving his index finger, a short stick, or lighting device 30–40 cm from the patient's eyes. The patient is asked to focus his eyes upon the tips of the moving object or light, with 10–20 movements as one session. 2 or 3 sessions may be performed per treatment. Move slowly initially, and then gradually increase the speed. Repeat the positive suggestions after each session.

After the above operation, the patient is asked to describe his feelings (whether the intrusive image, hallucination and scene has been darkened and how much; whether the color of painful emotion has lightened; and whether his confidence in his ability to adapt has increased) and also to briefly comment on the influence and effect of the treatment.

Modeling and Focus-shifting

In this approach, an appropriately positive psychological and behavioral model is set up by the therapist, which is repeatedly reinforced through life activity. The therapist can start conversations, play games, or participate in daily activities with the patient in order to subconsciously affect the patient with his own mental and behavioral well-being; even movies that show how people cope with life proactively after trauma can be helpful.

For PTSD patients, another commonly selected approach is focus-shifting. This refers to releasing the unpleasant emotions when they appear by singing, reading out loud, shouting, talking with friends, doing physical exercises, writing, and even crying loudly.

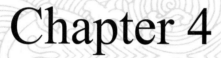

Chapter 4

PTSD Treatment—
Psychiatric and Integrative
Approaches

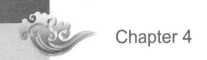

Diagnostic Criteria

The *Diagnostic and Statistical Manual of Mental Disorders* (*DSM-IV-TR*) classifies PTSD as an anxiety disorder. If symptoms last less than three months, the condition is diagnosed as *acute* PTSD. If symptoms last more than three months, it is considered *chronic* PTSD. The usual onset of symptoms is within six months of the traumatic event; otherwise, it is categorized as PTSD with *delayed onset*.

Diagnosis of PTSD

Re-experiencing (with one or more the following symptoms):

The traumatic patient is persistently re-experiencing recurrent and intrusive distressing recollections of the event, including images, thoughts, or perceptions, having recurrent distressing dreams of the event, acting or feeling as if the traumatic event were recurring (includes a sense of reliving the experience, illusions, hallucinations, and dissociative flashback episodes, including those that occur on awakening or when intoxicated), having intense psychological distress at exposure to internal or external cues that symbolize or resemble an aspect of the traumatic event, having physiological reactivity on exposure to internal or external cues that symbolize or resemble an aspect of the trauma.

Avoidance (with three or more of these symptoms):

Persistent efforts to avoid thoughts, activities, places, people, feelings, or conversations associated with the trauma. Patient has an inability to recall an important aspect of the trauma. Patient has markedly diminished interest or participation in significant activities. The trauma survivor feels detachment or estrangement from others. The patient feels "numb" on the inside (e.g., unable to have loving feelings). The trauma survivor senses a foreshortened future (e.g., does not expect to have a career, marriage, children or a normal life span).

Hyperarousal (Must have two or more of these symptoms):

Patient has difficulty falling or staying asleep. They are irritable and display frequent outbursts of anger. The trauma survivor has difficulty concentrating. They display symptoms of hypervigilance. They also exhibit exaggerated startle responses.

Duration of the disturbance (symptoms of re-experiencing, avoidance, hyperarousal) persists for more than one month. Additionally, the disturbance causes impairment in social, occupational, or other important areas of functioning.

Re-experiencing can take on different forms. The patient can have recurrent dreams about the event and dream-disturbed sleep frequented with nightmares relating to the experience. Patients also have psychological and physiological responses that remind them of the traumatic event (a location similar to where the event took place, an anniversary of the event, or sounds and smells that remind them of the event, etc.).

Patients with PTSD also function within an increased state of hyperarousal. These symptoms can include insomnia, irritability, outbursts of anger, difficulty concentrating, hypervigilance, and an exaggerated startled response. Patients often describe that they are "on edge" and cannot seem to relax.

Patients with PTSD display symptoms of avoidance. They will avoid places, people, or activities that remind them of the traumatic event. They may also appear "numb" and unable to express feelings towards their family and friends. Patients will describe that they feel "empty" on the inside. They may have an inability to recall important parts of the trauma. People with PTSD may become isolated and detached from others, lose interest in activities they used to enjoy, or have a restricted affect.

In addition to the DSM-IV, there are other psychological assessment tools that have been used to diagnose PTSD. The post-traumatic stress disorder checklist (PCL-M) is currently used in diagnosing military servicemembers. The PCL-M is a standardized, 17-item self-report measure of the DSM-IV symptoms of PTSD. Respondents also rate how much they were "bothered by the problem in the past month". Items are rated on a 5-point scale ranging from 1 ("not at all") to 5 ("extremely"). There are several versions of the PCL, with the original being the PCL-M (military). The PCL-M asks about problems in response to "stressful military experiences" instead of more generally about problems in relation to stressful experiences.

The Beck's Depression Inventory 2nd Edition (BDI-II) is often used in conjunction with the PCL-M to further assess the trauma survivor's depression severity levels. The BDI-II is standardized, self-reporting scale

for measuring symptoms of depression. The BDI-II consists of 21 items and is self-administered. Raw scores are converted to degrees of severity (i.e., 0-13 minimal, 14-19 mild, 20-28 moderate, 29-63 severe symptoms of depression). The BDI-2 was developed to assess depressive symptoms vis-à-vis DSM-IV. It has fair to good correlations (i.e., .68, .37, and .71) with other measures of depression (such as the Beck Hopelessness Scale, Suicide Probability Scale, and Revised Hamilton Psychiatric Rating Scale for Depression). Internal consistency (coefficient alpha) estimates of reliability range between .39 and .69, whereas the test-retest reliability estimate after one week is in the acceptable range (i.e., r = .93).

The Sheehan Disability Inventory (SDI) is also used often in conjunction with the PCL-M to measure the severity of impairments in social, occupational, or other important areas of functioning in PTSD patients. The SDI is a 3-item self-report scale measuring the severity of disability in the domains of work, family life/home responsibilities and social/leisure activities. Each of these three domains is scored on a ten-point Likert scale, where a score of 0 is 'not at all impaired', 5 is 'moderately impaired' and 10 is 'very severely impaired'. It provides a measure of total functional disability (range 0-30). It has been shown to have adequate internal reliability (α-coefficients and factor analyses) and construct/criterion related validity and has been used previously as an outcome measure in studies of PTSD and panic disorder.

The Clinician-Administered PTSD Scale (CAPS) is the gold standard in PTSD clinical assessment. The CAPS is a 30-item structured interview that corresponds to the DSM-IV criteria for PTSD. The CAPS can be used to make a current (past month) or lifetime diagnosis of PTSD or to assess symptoms over the previous week. In addition to assessing the 17 PTSD symptoms, questions target the impact of symptoms on social and occupational functioning, improvement in symptoms since a previous CAPS administration, overall response validity, overall PTSD severity, and frequency and intensity of five associated symptoms (guilt over acts, survivor guilt, gaps in awareness, depersonalization, and derealization). For each item, standardized questions and probes are provided. As part of the trauma assessment (Criterion A), the Life Events Checklist is used to identify traumatic stressors experienced. CAPS items are asked in reference to up to three traumatic stressors. The CAPS was designed to be administered by clinicians and clinical researchers who have a working knowledge of PTSD, but can also be administered by appropriately trained paraprofessionals.

The validity and reliability of the CAPS has proven to be adequate for assessment of posttraumatic stress disorder (PTSD) among military personnel. The Clinician-Administered PTSD Scale (CAPS) was given to 125 combat veterans, along with a computerized variant of the Structured Clinical Interview for DSM-Ⅲ-R for PTSD, the SCID-DTREE. (The SCID-DTREE was itself validated against the full SCID). Results showed the CAPS to be a good discriminator of PTSD: Out of the 125 cases, only 9 were misclassified using the SCID-DTREE as the base measure, a 93% efficiency. An alpha on the full CAPS was .95 This suggests that the CAPS is an appropriate scale for use with military combat veterans.

The Psychological Assessment Scale (PAS) is designed for use as a triage instrument within a health care system and is commonly used as in conjunction with the PCL-M, the DSM-IV Diagnostic Criteria for PTSD, and the Clinician-Administered PTSD Scale (CAPS) in the diagnosis of PTSD. The 22-item test will be used to assess distinct clinical domains, which are labeled Element scores. PAS Element scores include health problems, psychotic features, negative affect, acting out, social withdrawal, hostile control, alienation, anger control, alcohol problems, and suicidal thinking. The self-administered objective questionnaire was developed with reference to its parent instrument, the PAI. The reliability and validity of the PAS 22 items were determined through extensive item-analysis as the most sensitive to the broad range of contemporary clinical problems measured by the Personality Assessment Inventory (PAI). PAS reliability and validity scores were derived from normative data from a national community sample of 1000 adults matched for age, race and gender as well as for 1246 clinical participants and college students.

Psychiatric Treatment

The treatment standard for PTSD mainly utilizes cognitive-behavioral therapy and pharmacotherapy. Cognitive-behavioral therapy comprises of two forms of psychotherapy that includes cognitive therapy and exposure therapy. Cognitive therapy mainly identifies thoughts about the world and oneself that are making you feel afraid or upset. Patients will learn to replace these thoughts with more accurate and less distressing thoughts. Cognitive therapy helps you understand that the traumatic event you lived through was not your fault. In exposure therapy, the goal is to have less fear about your memories through repeated imagination or in person confrontations of feared stimuli. Systematic desensitization is one form of exposure therapy where the patient repeatedly imagines weak-anxiety-arousing stimulus until stimulus loses ability to evoke anxiety (Wilson 2004).

Antidepressants, mainly the Selective Serotonin Reuptake Inhibitors (SSRIs) are the first-line pharmaceutical agents recommended for the treatment of PTSD, [5] however many classes of medications have been used off label for PTSD for several years. These include Serotonin/Norepinephrine Reuptake Inhibitors (SNRIs), Tricyclic Antidepressants (TCAs) Monoamine Oxidase Inhibitors (MAOIs), Atypical Antipsychotics, Benzodiazepines, Adrenergic-Inhibiting Agents, and Anticonvulsants. Other agents such as trazodone, bupropion (Wellbutrin SR/XL), and mirtazapine (Remeron®) have limited or inconclusive data in association with PTSD, so their use is not currently recommended.[5]

Selective Serotonin Reuptake Inhibitors (SSRI)

Sertraline (Zoloft®) and paroxetine (Paxil®) were the first two FDA approved SSRIs for the treatment of PTSD, but all SSRIs are considered equally efficacious.[5] Fluoxetine (Prozac®) was one of the first SSRIs to be widely marketed and used for anxiety disorders (including PTSD) and others include Citalopram (Celxa®), escitalopram (Lexapro®), fluvoxamine (Luvox®) and zimelidine (Zelmid®). SSRIs increase the extracellular level of the neurotransmitter serotonin by inhibiting its reuptake into the presynaptic cell, increasing the level of serotonin available to bind with the postsynaptic receptor. They have varying degrees of selectivity for the other monoamine transporters, with pure SSRIs having only weak affinity for the noradrenaline and dopamine transporter. Increasing serotonin levels in the brain via this mechanism is thought to improve mood and lessen anxiety states (please refer to later chapters in this book describing the theorized biological mechanism for this effect). Several large placebo-controlled trials showed that several of the SSRIs had twice the success rate than placebo in ameliorating PTSD symptoms[6-8] at four to six weeks of treatment, however some studies suggest a course of six to nine months of treatment before observing full benefits.[5,9] Common side effects include dry mouth, nausea, sexual dysfunction, drowsiness, gastrointenstinal distress and if the side effects render them intolerable or high doses have no response, the below agents should be considered.

Serotonin Norsepinephrine Reuptake Inhibitors (SNRIs)

SNRIs act upon and increase the levels of two neurotransmitters in the brain that are known to play an important part in mood, these being serotonin and norepinephrine. There are several SNRIs on the market but the only one (venlafaxine/Effexor XR®) to date was tested in a double-blind study for PTSD.[10] At moderate doses (>150mg/day) it acts on serotonergic and noradrenergic systems, whereas at high doses (>300mg/day) it also affects dopaminergic neurotransmission. One study showed it was venlafaxine was equally efficacious and tolerable as sertraline for the treatment of PTSD symptoms[10] but anecdotally venlafaxine has long been used to target anxiety and depressive symptoms equally.

Tricyclic Antidepressants (TCAs) and Monoamine Oxidase Inhibitors (MAOIs)

The TCAs are the oldest, cheapest, and most studied of all the FDA approved antidepressants available on the market, and the MAOIs the most efficacious for mood disorders; however the MAOIs dietary restrictions and potential for severe side effects limits their usage. The TCAs Amitriptyline, phenelzine, and imipramine have shown promise like the SSRIs in controlling PTSD, however they are often not used due to their anticholinergic (sedating) and cardiovascular side effects. One study indicated that SSRIs were superior to treating symptoms than TCAs, however Imipramine was the most successful TCAs in this study,[11] but both classes of agents are considered second or third-line agents restricted to resistant cases.[5]

Atypical Antipsychotics

The atypical antipsychotics (also known as second generation antipsychotics) are a group of antipsychotic drugs used to treat psychiatric

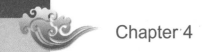

conditions. Some atypical antipsychotics are FDA approved for use in the treatment of schizophrenia. Some carry FDA approved indications for acute mania, bipolar mania, psychotic agitation, bipolar maintenance, and other indications. The atypicals are a group of unrelated drugs united by the fact that they work differently from typical antipsychotics. Most share a common attribute of working on serotonin receptors as well as dopamine receptors, however some work solely on partial dopamine partial agonism. Atypical antipsychotics were effective as monotherapy and as adjunctive therapy to SSRIs in open-label, small double-blind, placebo-controlled trials, and case studies. Atypicals are mainly considered in PTSD where paranoia or flashbacks are prominent, and in lower doses to augment SSRIs treatment where montherapy with an SSRI has breakthrough symptoms.[12] Riseridone (Risperdal®), olanzapine (Zyprexa®), ziprasidone (Geodon®), aripiprazole (Abilify®) and quetiapine (Seroquel®) have all been documented in the medical literature for off-label usage for severe PTSD symptoms refractory to monotherapy SSRI treatment, however specific studies have focused mainly on risperidone,[13] olanzapine,[14] and quetiapine.[15] At times, an atypical antipsychotic may be useful as monotherapy,[16] however this class of medication is mainly recommended ad adjunctive treatment to SSRI therapy and that patients be well educated about the side effects of their use (hyperglycemia, weight gain, increased appetite, lipid abnormalities, and extrapyramidal symptoms).[5]

Benzodiazepines

Benzodiazepines enhance the effect of the neurotransmitter gamma-aminobutyric acid, which results in sedative, hypnotic (sleep-inducing), anxiolytic (anti-anxiety), anticonvulsant (anti-seizure), muscle relaxant and amnesic actions. These properties make benzodiazepines useful in treating insomnia, anxiety, seizures, muscle spasms, agitation and alcohol withdrawal. Benzodiazepines are categorized as either short-, intermediate- or long-acting. Short- and intermediate-acting benzodiazepines are preferred for the treatment of insomnia; longer-acting benzodiazepines are recommended for the treatment of anxiety. Benzodiazepines have been found to be ineffective in a double-blind, placebo-controlled study but had been used based on case reports indicating positive results with their use.[12] Many clinicians either avoid this class or used them short term because of potential depressive side effects, and the possibility that PTSD may worsen with long term use.[12] The benzodiazepines have addictive potential as well, however anecdotally they have been used short term to help patients tolerate the increased agitation that can occur with initiating SSRI therapy, which commonly occurs with the PTSD population.[17] The most commonly used long acting benzodiazepines for PTSD are clonazepam (Klonopin®) and diazepam (Valium®). Medium half-life benzodiazepines include Lorazepam (Ativan®) and temazepam (Restoril®), and alprazolam (Xanax®) is the most commonly used short acting benzodiazepine.[17]

Adrenergic-Inhibiting Agents

This class of medication is rarely used as monotherapy. The most commonly used medications in this class used for adjunctive therapy include Prazosin (Minpress®, an alpha-1 receptor antagonist) and propranolol (Inderal®, a beta blocker).[5] PTSD patients have been shown to have hyperactivity of their central nervous system (CNS) norepinephrine centers in their brains.[18] Clinical trials have shown that Prazosin improve nighttime arousal (sleep disturbance) and re-experiencing symptoms (nightmare), however daytime dosing has also been studied and shown to suppress autonomic arousal related to traumatic cues[19] (Taylor, Biol Psychiatry). Propranolol are usually taken to prevent the symptoms of PTSD by blocking postsynaptic norepinephrine receptors, and studies have shown that patients taking beta blockers have decreased physiological responses to reminders of their trauma.[20,21]

Anticonvulsants

Anticonvulsants are normally used for the treatment of seizures but have been found to have mood stabilizing effects. The goal of an anticonvulsant is to suppress the rapid and excessive firing of neurons that start a seizure. Because of this, anticonvulsants also have proven effective in treating many kinds of dysfunctional anxiety. In psychiatric practice, they are mostly used for the treatment of bipolar disorder, however patients with co-morbid PTSD have reported reduction in their PTSD symptoms.[5] The major molecular targets of marketed anticonvulsant drugs are voltage-gated sodium channels, components of the GABA system, and

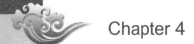

voltage-gated calcium channels. Carbamazepine (Tegretol®) studied in an open label trial decreased re-experiencing symptoms and insomnia,[22] while Valproic Acid (Depakote®) decreased arousal and avoidance symptoms.[23] Both these anticonvulsants have significant side-effects and require frequent monitoring, which affects patient compliance and a providers willingness to prescribe them. Topiramate (Topamax®) and Gabapentin (Neurontin®) have shown some promise in small studies and have less side effects however further studies need to be done to assess their full potential as adjunctive therapy.[5] Lamotrigine (Lamictal®) is usually used for depressive phases of bipolar illness due to its mood elevating effects, however a small double-blind trial showed promise for improving re-experiencing and emotional numbing.[24]

Conclusion

PTSD is a complex psychiatric disorder with several pharmacological interventions available to prescribers. Pharmacotherapy attempts to target the core symptoms that predominate the clinical presentation (re-experiencing, arousal and avoidance symptoms) and antidepressants, specifically the SSRIs, are considered first-line treatment, followed by SNRIs and adjunctive atypical antipsychotic/andrenergic-inhibiting agents. Anticonvulsants show promise but need to be studied further, and TCAs/MAOIs are considered third line treatment. Short term benzodiazepine usage (preferably long acting) is controversial at worst, with long term use strongly discouraged.

Integrative Treatment

The initiatives at the U.S. Army occurred mainly because traditional methods of treating PTSD weren't long enough in duration, weren't intense enough or comprehensive enough. So an integrative PTSD program was created at William Beaumont Army Medical Center that would address all aspects of PTSD and treat the "whole soldier". This integrative approach treats many of the symptoms of PTSD that are not addressed through the standard mental health protocols that included cognitive-behavioral therapy and pharmacotherapy. The integrative approaches at these programs incorporated the integration of massage therapy, pool therapy, expressive art therapy, meditation, yoga, acupuncture, marital/family therapy, as well as Reiki energy work combined with the standard treatment protocols of cognitive-behavioral and cathartic psychotherapies and pharmacotherapy.

Standard behavioral health approach tends to medicate the central nervous system, which leads to changes in cognition, emotion, and behavior. Additionally, psychotherapy is utilized to help cope with symptoms. This treatment approach mostly treats from the inside out. The goal is to manage physiological symptoms of PTSD (i.e., hyperarousal, anxiety, insomnia, panic attacks, depression).

Alternative medical effect intervenes physiologically to reduce arousal through the movement qi and energy leading to changes in cognition, emotion, and behavior.

There tends to be a cumulative effect leading to physiological changes (i.e., melatonin, cortisol, fMRI neuronal signal reduction in the limbic system) and reduction in hypertonicity and hyperarousal.

When you integrate both Western and Eastern modalities, this provides a good synergistic approach. Western standard mental health methods (pharmacotherapy and cognitive-behavioral therapy) can resolve about sixty percent of the symptoms of PTSD. But what do you do with the other forty percent of the residual symptoms of PTSD? It is my experience that the utilization of Eastern modalities provides the best approach when utilized in conjunction with Western mental health methods. Typically, on any given day at the Ft. Bliss Restoration & Resilience Center at William Beaumont Army Medical Center, soldiers go through group and individual counseling and in addition, utilize pharmacotherapy to manage their pain, insomnia, depression, traumatic brain injury headaches, anxiety, and panic attacks. Soldiers then go through biofeedback, Reiki, yoga, tai-chi, acupuncture, and medical massage for the remaining residual symptoms of PTSD.

Typically, alternative modalities can be used in combinatorial approaches for the residual symptoms of PTSD. For example, medical massage and acupuncture can be utilized for pain management, for the reduction of physical arousal, and reduction in hyperarousal. In a combinatorial approach, medical massage can be used with acupuncture for the reduction of physical arousal. Soldiers typically display muscular hypertonicity that can cause muscular pain localized

in the trapezius, SCM, and the upper and lower back. Medical massage and acupuncture can help resolve this medical condition through deep tissue massage techniques and through local trigger points to release muscular tension. The same approach can be used to treat pain through the treatment of shoulder, knee, and back pain with deep tissue massage techniques and with localized trigger points to reduce pain in these areas. For hyperarousal symptoms (i.e., anxiety, stress, insomnia, and anger) treatment is mainly focused on the treatment of the back. Soldiers who have gone through multiple traumas in combat tends to hold their anxiety and stress in their back, mostly in their trapezius, GB channel, and upper and lower back, BL channel. The reduction of hyperarousal can be easily obtained through the treatment of these localized areas.

The combinatorial approach of Reiki and acupuncture is best used in the treatment of insomnia and anxiety. Typically, acupuncture sessions should occur in conjunction with Reiki treatments.

Acupuncture needles should be placed at GB 21 (*jiān jǐng*), SP 6 (*sān yīn jiāo*), ST 36 (*zú sān lǐ*), LI 4 (*hé gǔ*), *yìn táng* (EX-HN3) and DU 20 (*bǎi huì*) with the client in a supine position. Reiki treatments can then occur while the acupuncture needles are retained for 20 minutes above these acupoints.

The patient can tend be treated in a prone position with these acupoints: GB 20 (*fēng chí*), HT 3 (*shào hǎi*), BL 15 (*xīn shù*), BL 16 (*dū shù*), BL 18 (*gān shù*), BL 19 (*dǎn shù*), BL 20 (*pí shù*), BL 23 (*shèn shù*). Reiki treatments can then occur while the acupuncture needles are retained for 40 minutes.

The combinatorial approach of biofeedback and acupuncture is best used in the treatment of insomnia and anxiety. Typically, acupuncture sessions should occur in conjunction with biofeedback treatments.

Acupuncture needles should be placed on GB 21 (*jiān jǐng*), SP 6 (*sān yīn jiāo*), ST 36 (*zú sān lǐ*), LI 4 (*hé gǔ*), and ear points *shenmen*, *yìn táng* (EX-HN3) and DU 20 (*bǎi huì*). Biofeedback sessions can then occur while the acupuncture needles are retained for 60 minutes.

So far, there are four comprehensive post-traumatic stress disorder (PTSD) and combat stress treatment programs in the U.S. Army that have incorporated different complementary and alternative medicine approaches in their treatment programs. Many of these comprehensive programs started as a result of the program at the Ft. Bliss Restoration & Resilience Center.

The initiatives at the Ft. Bliss Restoration & Resilience Center occurred through strong advocates that supported the integrated approach in the treatment of PTSD. Advocates at Ft. Bliss wanted an integrated program that utilized western mental health protocols along with complementary and alternative modalities. So, a program was created that would address all aspects of PTSD and treat the "whole soldier". This integrative approach treats man of the symptoms of PTSD that are not addressed through the standard mental health protocols that included cognitive-behavioral therapy and pharmacotherapy.

At the Ft. Bliss Restoration & Resilience Center, the intensive six-month program utilizes a holistic approach in the treatment of PTSD. The treatment program is a comprehensive holistic approach that uses psychotherapy, group therapy, Reiki, medical massage, acupuncture, yoga, Tai chi, and meditation. Additionally, there is a physical component in this program. Soldiers go through a daily 45-minute "power walk" and they also play water polo three times a week.

Theoretical Foundation

The Ft. Bliss Restoration & Resilience Center treatment framework of traumatic stress is based on a current understanding of the neurobiology of stress and trauma. Our nervous system is built to react to a traumatic event through automated responses in the sympathetic nervous system. In times of heightened stress, our system will go through a series of responses triggered by catecholamine hormones. There will be an acceleration of heart and lung action, gastrointestinal inhibition, constriction of blood vessels, dilation of the pupils, auditory exclusion, and a loss of peripheral vision.

The nervous system is designed to react and then recover from stressful or traumatic events. After a traumatic incident, our system slows down and a series of responses kick in order to restore the body to a homeostatic state. The heart rate slows, blood vessels dilate, and pupils constrict. In short, we move from an output of high energy to a relatively

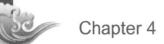

settled and balanced state. This is the natural response of the nervous system to traumatic stress.

In terms of Chinese medicine and how it correlates to the modern neurobiology of traumatic stress, there is a link between the sympathetic system and the various channels in Chinese medicine. First, during traumatic stress there is one main channel affected by the traumatic event: the heart. The heart governs the mind and consciousness, and it also presides over the other viscera. When dysfunction of the heart occurs after long periods of traumatic stress, other channels also become dysfunctional with the liver, spleen, and kidney channels being most often involved. Symptoms of anger and irritability indicate that liver qi is stagnant. Feeling uncentered, ungrounded, and with melancholy shows an imbalance of spleen-earth. Insomnia, loss of memory, and low back are associated with non-communication of heart and kidney.

Yet, people who have experienced traumatic stress may operate with their presence and energy in a state of hyperarousal and hypervigilance, or in a disconnected and depressed state. They cannot seem to function within a state of equilibrium; they are either functioning with high energy levels and high psychomotor discharge (anxiety, agitated, panic attacks, hypervigilant, insomnia) or they are functioning with low energy levels (depression, disconnected, disassociated). People who have experienced traumatic stress will fluctuate between a high state of energy and an extremely low state of energy.

The integrative approach at the Ft. Bliss Restoration & Resilience Center utilizes both Western approaches (i.e., pharmacotherapy, cognitive processing therapy) and alternative modalities such as Chinese Medicine, acupuncture, Reiki, and medical massage to stabilize our soldiers both physically, mentally, and spiritually.

FT. BLISS RESTORATION & RESILIENCE CENTER: TREATMENT FRAMEWORK

1) AGORAPHOBIA/CLAUSTROPHOBIA REDUCTION TRACK
Goal: Increase tolerance for public places, crowds, enclosed areas
Interventions: Therapeutic outings to challenging public places (malls, bowling alleys, Carlsbad Caverns)

2) COGNITIVE-BEHAVIOR TRACK

Goal: Reduce cognitive distortions and errors related to combat experience

Intervention(s): Individual and group psychotherapy with CBT interventions

3) COGNITIVE REHABILITATION TRACK

Goal: Reduce hyperarousal to increase ability to focus and attend, and improve memory functioning (encoding and retrieval) through hippocampal rehabilitation

Intervention(s):

- *Hyperarousal reduction*: Acupuncture, biofeedback, Reiki, medical massage, daily power walk, daily physical training, water polo, and movement therapies (tai-chi, qi-gong, yoga)
- *Improvement in Memory Functioning*: Brain train (computer-based cognitive rehabilitation program)

4) EMOTIONAL/GRIEF WORK TRACK

Goal: Reduce negative emotional valence attached to distressing combat memories/images

Intervention(s): Individual and group psychotherapy, expressive (art) therapy focused on emotional processing and grief work

5) MILITARY REINTEGRATION TRACK

Goal: Increase ability to tolerate combat-simulated environments and activities

Interventions: Engagement Skills Trainer (EST) 2000 (indoor simulated firing range); brief group missions (day-long Habitat for Humanity mission)

Planned: Live range firing, shooting houses, IED lane, week-long Habitat for Humanity mission

6) PHYSICAL AROUSAL REDUCTION TRACK

Goal: Reduce physical agitation, startle response, muscular hypertonicity

Interventions: Acupuncture, biofeedback, Reiki, medical massage, daily power walk, daily physical training, water polo, and movement

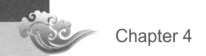

therapies (Tai-chi, Qi-gong, Yoga)

7) RE-SOCIALIZATION TRACK

Goal: Increase tolerance for/ability to engage in social interaction with comrades, friends, family

Interventions: Recreation room, therapeutic outings (planetarium, golf, bumper cars, water polo, social events)

8) SPIRITUAL (META-COGNITIVE) HEALING TRACK

Goal: Help achieve a cohesive, reliable, robust self-image, re-conceptualize a "meaning" for their lives, work through issues of death and dying, and (if appropriate) develop a more mature concept of deity that can be "squared" with their combat experience.

Interventions: Individual/group psychotherapy, counseling with a facility chaplain, cross-cultural group experiences (Native American sweat lodge, etc.)

The comprehensive PTSD and combat stress treatment programs that have started as a result of the program at Ft. Bliss are listed below:

At the Warrior Combat Stress Reset Program at Ft. Hood, their intensive combat stress three-week program focuses on the reduction of hyperarousal and reactivity. Reducing these core symptoms of combat stress and post-traumatic stress disorder allows other treatments to be more effective. The program includes group counseling, biofeedback, individual counseling, and alternative therapies (massage, acupuncture, yoga, Reiki).

The Deployment Health Clinical Center at Walter Reed Army Medical Center uses evidence-based therapies in a comprehensive three-week program. Soldiers learn coping skills to reduce intrusive symptoms like hyperarousal and avoidance. The program also provides a therapeutic group process for mutual support and re-integration into family and community. Additionally, soldiers are taught stress management and practice various forms of relaxation (guided imagery, yoga, progressive muscle relaxation, deep abdominal breathing).

The Landstuhl Regional Medical Center uses an intensive eight-week therapeutic post-traumatic stress disorder day treatment program that includes a holistic approach. During the eight-hour days, patients will participate in multiple disciplines and interests, including art therapy, yoga and meditation classes, substance abuse groups, anger and grief management, tobacco cessation, pain management and multiple PTSD evidence-based practice protocols. The evidence-based practice protocols include eye movement desensitization and reprocessing (EMDR), cognitive processing therapy, and prolonged exposure therapy.

Most of these comprehensive programs have three main components in their treatment programs: cognitive disturbance resolution, functional ability improvement, and affect and behavior dysregulation resolution.

Affect and Behavior Dysregulation Resolution

Issues with self-harm, suicidal ideation and homicidal ideation are all due to problems of dysregulation. Additional problems with depression, hyperarousal, and hypervigilance are also attributed to affect and behavior dysregulation.

In a study by Yehuda et al. (1996), researchers found that PTSD patients exhibited lower base levels of cortisol than normal subjects, leaving adrenaline to run freely throughout the body during trauma. Adrenaline aids in the imprint of strong emotional events, while cortisol helps keep adrenaline in check. Thus, a patient with lower base levels of cortisol would more likely form a strong memory of the trauma. PTSD patients also display atypical brainwave activity, reduction in the size of the hippocampus, over-activation of the amygdala, excessive arousal of the sympathetic nervous system (i.e., stress response), and higher levels of endogenous opiates (e.g., endorphins).

The treatment frameworks in more comprehensive programs utilize pharmacotherapy in concert with alternative modalities such as acupuncture, Reiki, yoga, meditation, biofeedback, and tai-chi to effectively regulate hyperarousal symptoms of PTSD and the enhanced sympathetic response.

Cognitive Disturbance Resolution

Researchers have found that dysfunctional family systems and prolonged childhood abuse also result in cognitive disturbances in most trauma survivors. According to Dr. Mungadze from Dallas Baptist University, "Deficiencies in childhood development such as inconsistent parenting, interpersonal conflict, lack of encouragement and warmth, and gross neglect have been found to contribute significantly to adult psychopathology. These environmental deficiencies undermine the development of healthy attachments and a secure sense of self."

Trauma survivors who were severely traumatized as children grow into adults who already live in a state of hyperarousal. According to Dr. Schiraldi in his book, *The Post-Traumatic Stress Disorder Resource Book*, "Trauma survivors tend to utilize dissociation as a defense against distressful and painful experiences. The mind walls off trauma to try to contain it in much the same way as the body walls off infection. Dissociation can be regarded as a coping mechanism. As long as we wall off the painful experience, we gain protection. Dissociation enables the preexisting personality to sense that it has been preserved and can carry on."

With multiple traumas experienced during childhood or as an adult, each trauma tends to become compartmentalized. Comprehensive treatment programs also utilize cognitive therapy to resolve the cognitive disturbances (negative beliefs about oneself) brought about by trauma. Psycho-education groups and cognitive restructuring techniques help these patients to confront and dispute their cognitive distortions.

Functional Ability Improvement

Psychopathology causes deterioration in a patient's functional ability, and part of a comprehensive program involves the teaching of healthy coping skills that enable a patient to improve their quality of life independently.

These tools help the survivor to relate more effectively to those around them, become a better family member, and to overcome many of the obstacles in handling anxiety, social situations, self-esteem issues. Breathing techniques, meditation, sleep hygiene, psycho-education groups, Emotional Freedom Technique (EFT), and Cranial Electrical Stimulation (CES) devices can all be used as tools for such patients.

Teaching the survivor to make significant changes in their dysfunctional behaviors (i.e., drugs, alcohol, sex, or self-harming behaviors) is essential for maintaining functional ability. Instead of taking responsibility and owning their experiences, PTSD survivors tend to minimize and avoid them. For some, looking at the trauma and learning new coping skills in order to function in everyday life is very difficult, and dissociation is an easier way for them to cope.

Steps to Recovery

Recovery unfolds in three stages. The first stage involves the establishment of individual safety. The central task of the second stage is remembrance and mourning. The central task of the third stage is reconnection with ordinary life.

Again, the first task of recovery is to effectively establish the survivor's safety. No other therapeutic work should even be attempted until a reasonable degree of safety has been achieved. Survivors feel as if they cannot control their physical bodies; they may even feel as if someone else is controlling them. Their emotions and their thinking feel out of control, they feel unsafe in relation to other people, and are often afraid that they will have an explosive reaction when others are around them. They feel both unsafe and "out of control" within their own environment. The strategies of therapy must address the patient's safety concerns in all of these domains.

The physical symptoms of post-traumatic stress disorder can be modified with physical strategies that will help to change the hyperarousal aspect of the disorder. These include the use of medications to reduce reactivity and hyperarousal, and also the use of techniques to modulate the sympathetic nervous system such as relaxation, vigorous exercise, acupuncture, Reiki, massage therapy, and biofeedback.

The mental confusion associated the disorder can be addressed with cognitive and behavioral strategies. These include recognition and naming of symptoms, the use of daily logs to chart symptoms and adaptive responses, and cognitive behavioral therapy.

The destruction of attachments that occur with the disorder must be addressed by interpersonal strategies which include the gradual development of trusting relationships in individual and group psychotherapy.

Finally, the social alienation must be addressed through social strategies by mobilizing the survivor's natural support systems of family members, friends, and spouses. Once a sense of safety has been established, environmental safety issues are addressed with individual and group education. These environmental issues include the establishment of a safe living situation, as well as the establishment of a secure financial plan.

In the second stage of recovery, the survivor tells the story of the trauma, recounted completely and in great detail. In many instances, a traumatic survivor will compartmentalize and dissociate from their traumatic memories in order to survive. The reconstruction process will begin by recovering their fragmented memories and gradually integrating them into their current memory. Recitation of the facts and reconstruction of the trauma should also include the survivor's interpretation of the meaning of the event.

The telling of the traumatic story will be a difficult process, because the survivor will experience extreme grief. However, this mourning process is the most crucial part of the healing process, because patients often feel as if they are stuck in time. Some describe the grief and mourning as if a faucet has been opened, where a seemingly endless stream of water and tears flow constantly. This process of repeated recitation of the traumatic event, eventually bears fruit, where memories become less vivid and emotional attachment to the pain and darkness of the traumatic event begin to fade.

The central task of the third stage is reconnection, because trauma tends to have an isolating effect on the individual. Survivors detach themselves from the outside world, and isolate themselves from others. Reconnecting with the outside world is another important step, and these crucial bonds are often formed in therapeutic group settings.

During group psychotherapy, survivors begin to feel that they are not alone and that they have nothing to be ashamed of; there is no stigma or judgment because they are simply in a group amongst their peers. Nowhere is this healing experience more powerful than within a group.

Compassion Fatigue

Compassion fatigue is a term that refers to a gradual lessening of compassion over time. Healthcare providers exhibit several symptoms including hopelessness, a decrease in experiences of pleasure, constant stress and anxiety, and a pervasive negative attitude.

This can have detrimental effects on individuals, both professionally and personally, including a decrease in productivity, the inability to focus, and the development of new feelings of incompetence and self-doubt.

Compassion fatigue affects three main viscera: liver, heart, and kidney. When there is qi deficiency, the practitioner will first experience fatigue, often followed by other symptoms associated with the affected viscus. Constant exposure to trauma first affects the kidney, so healthcare providers who are under constant exposure to trauma patients, will first feel fatigued with an inability to focus and also a perceived decrease in experiences of pleasure. From a TCM perspective, such symptoms are mainly associated with kidney deficiency.

The second viscus affected is the liver. When there is qi deficiency involving the kidney, liver qi will also stagnate. Qi stagnation leads to an unsmooth flow of qi which can result in stress. Associated symptoms will include a pervasive negative attitude as well as anger and frustration.

The third viscus affected is the heart. When there is liver qi stagnation, the free flow of qi to the heart is also impaired. Furthermore, when qi becomes deficient, blood deficiency often follows. In that case, with not enough blood to nourish the heart, the heart becomes disturbed and anxiety results.

Chapter 5
Acupuncture Treatment

PTSD Acupuncture Protocol at the Ft. Bliss Restoration & Resilience Center

The acupuncture protocol utilized by the integrative PTSD program at the Ft. Bliss Restoration & Resilience Center involves a standard acupuncture point prescription for treatment of the three main viscera affected by PTSD: the heart, spleen, and liver. Specifically, this protocol utilizes points to reduce the main symptoms of PTSD (i.e., hyperarousal, hypertonicity, anxiety, depression, and insomnia) by calming the spirit, tonifying spleen qi and promoting the free movement of liver qi. The standard acupuncture protocol combines front and back treatments to avoid point fatigue or tolerance due to frequent use.

- Back treatments include the following acupuncture points needled bilaterally:

BL 15 (*xīn shù*), BL 16 (*dū shù*), BL 18 (*gān shù*), BL 19 (*dǎn shù*), BL 20 (*pí shù*), BL 23 (*shèn shù*), GB 20 (*fēng chí*), GB 21 (*jiān jǐng*), HT 3 (*shào hǎi*).

All needles are retained for 40 minutes.

- Front-body acupuncture points: LI 4 (*hé gǔ*), ST 36 (*zú sān lǐ*), SP 6 (*sān yīn jiāo*), LV 3 (*tài chōng*), and *yìn táng* (EX-HN3), DU 20 (*bǎi huì*), *sì shén cōng* (EX-HN1).

Five points on the outer BL line can also be alternated with their corresponding back-*shu* points at the inner BL line. Their names clearly relate to the mental-spiritual aspects of the relevant yin organ:

Lung *shu* point: BL 13 (*fèi shù*)
Pò—Corporeal soul
BL 42 (*pò hù*)—Corporeal soul door (for grief)

Heart *shu* point: BL 15 (*xīn shù*)
Shen—Spirit
BL 44 (*shén táng*)—Spirit hall (for excess joy)

Liver *shu* point: BL 18 (*gān shù*)
Hún—Ethereal soul
BL 47 (*hún mén*)—Door to the ethereal soul (for anger)

Spleen *shu* point: BL 20 (*pí shù*)

Yì—Reflection

BL 49 (*yì shè*)—House of reflection (for rumination, worry)

Kidney *shu* point: BL 23 (*shèn shù*)

Zhì—Will

BL 52 (*zhì shì*)—Room of the will (for fear)

All needles are inserted to a depth of ¼ to ½ inch. Manipulation techniques are employed according to the presenting pattern and patient constitution.

Moving cupping is then applied on the first line of the BL channel from BL 13 (*fèi shù*) to BL 25 (*dà cháng shù*) to reduce muscular tension and hypertonicity.

After each treatment, vaccaria seeds are also placed at ear points *Shenmen*, Heart, Nervous Subcortex, Sympathetic, Kidney, and Neurasthenia areas. All six auricular points are used, three in each ear. Patients are instructed to massage each point for at least 10 minutes per day for one week as part of their home-based therapy.

During the acute stage, the heart and the liver are generally affected, often accompanied by the presence of internal heat. These patients will display frequent panic attacks, anger, nightmares, insomnia, palpitations, difficulty breathing, and left arm numbness.

In the chronic stage, the kidney, spleen, and heart are affected. Patients will display fatigue, memory loss, insomnia, depression, sexual dysfunction, and a lack of desire for normal activities.

Modifications

After five treatments with the standard protocol, the following modifications may be applied in accordance with the presenting signs and symptoms:

> ➢ With predominant irritability and anger, add LV 2 (*xíng jiān*), four gates [*hé gǔ* (LI 4) and *tài chōng* (LV 3)], ear point Liver.
> ➢ With frequent insomnia, add points *Anmian*, ST 36 (*zú sān lǐ*), SP 6 (*sān yīn jiāo*), KI 3 (*tài xī*), KI 6 (*zhào hǎi*).
> ➢ With predominant night terrors and nightmares, add HT 5 (*tōng*

73

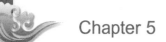

lǐ), HT 7 (*shén mén*), PC 6 (*nèi guān*), ear point Heart.

➢ With predominant depression, apply electro-acupuncture to acupoint pairs BL 15 (*xīn shù*) / BL 16 (*dū shù*), BL 18 (*gān shù*) / BL 23 (*shèn shù*), or *sì shén cōng* (EX-HN1) / DU 20 (*bǎi huì*).

PTSD and Five-phase Acupuncture

The Five-phase theory consists of a generation cycle and a restraining cycle. The generation cycle includes the following relationships:

* Wood feeds Fire
* Fire creates Earth
* Earth bears Metal
* Metal contains Water
* Water nourishes Wood

The restraining cycle includes the following:

* Wood parts Earth
* Earth absorbs Water
* Water quenches Fire
* Fire melts Metal
* Metal cuts Wood

When examining a symptom checklist for PTSD, many of the typical symptoms will also correlate to disharmonies of liver-wood, kidney-water, and heart-fire:

➢ Repeated disturbing dreams correlate to a heart imbalance. (Fire)

➢ Angry outbursts and irritability correlate to a liver imbalance. (Wood)

➢ Feeling severely distressed also correlates to a liver imbalance. (Wood)

➢ Repeated disturbing memories and thoughts correlate to a kidney imbalance. (Water)

➢ Trouble falling or staying asleep correlates to a heart and kidney imbalance. (Fire/Water)

➢ Being easily startled correlates to a heart imbalance. (Fire)

➢ Feeling emotionally numb correlates to a heart imbalance. (Fire)

➢ Being "super alert" also correlates to a heart imbalance. (Fire)

Therefore, treatments utilizing five-phase acupuncture for PTSD should focus on two of the restraining cycles:

- Water restrains Fire
- Metal restrains Wood

Of particular importance are the points on the Large Intestine channel and the Urinary Bladder channel. BL channel points are selected to reduce excessive qi associated with the heart, liver, and pericardium. Select BL 15 (*xīn shù*), BL 16 (*dū shù*), BL 18 (*gān shù*), and BL 19 (*dǎn shù*).

Also needle BL 23 (*shèn shù*) with supplementation to enhance the restraining effect of the water-phase on the fire-phase. Kidney points such as KI 3 (*tài xī*) and KI 6 (*zhào hǎi*) can be added for an additive restraining effect.

Large Intestine channel points are selected to reduce the effects of the wood-phase, particularly the liver channel. Select LI 4 (*hé gǔ*), LI 11 (*qū chí*).

Liver channel points are selected to reduce liver qi and promote the free flow of qi. Select LV 2 (*xíng jiān*), LV 3 (*tài chōng*).

Once wood and fire phases have returned to balance, the earth phase should be addressed in order to strengthen the movement of qi within the water phase. Water acts to anchor internal heat that will typically rise upward to disquiet the heart-spirit. When the symptoms of PTSD are associated with deficiencies of qi and blood, earth-points can be especially nourishing; they also help to promote the free flow of liver qi and calm the heart. Select SP 6 (*sān yīn jiāo*), SP 10 (*xuè hǎi*), ST 36 (*zú sān lǐ*).

Sun Si-miao Ghost Points

PTSD patients often suffer with insomnia, dream-disturbed sleep, nightmares, and repeated disturbing memories, thoughts, and images of their traumatic event. In soldiers, many of these distressing memories can involve the death of a comrade during war or traumatic images of rape, or torture. Ghost points are helpful and effective for reducing these disturbing memories and dreams.

The protocol includes needling of the following ghost points, which are actually a group of thirteen experiential points indicated for mental disease, insanity, and severe emotional depression.

For each session, select a group of three different points. Puncture or

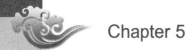

prick to bleed.

- LU 11 (*shào shāng*) Lesser Shang
  Jing-Well & Wood Point
- LI 11 (*qū chí*) Pool at the Bend
  He-Sea & Earth Point
  Ma Dan-yang Heavenly Star Point
- ST 6 (*jiá chē*) Jawbone
- SP 1 (*yǐn bái*) Hidden White
  Jing-well & Wood Point
- BL 62 (*shēn mài*) Extending Vessel
  Confluent Point of the Yang Motility Vessel
- PC 7 (*dà líng*) Great Mound
  Yuan-source Point
  Shu-stream & Earth Point
- PC 8 (*láo gōng*) Palace of Toil
  Ying-spring & Fire Point
- RN 1 (*huì yīn*) Meeting of Yin
  Meeting Point of the Conception, Penetrating, and Governing Vessels
- RN 24 (*chéng jiāng*) Sauce Receptacle
  Meeting Point of the Conception and Governing Vessels and the Large Intestine and Stomach Channels
- DU 16 (*fēng fǔ*) Wind Mansion
  -Point of the Sea of Marrow, Meeting Point of the Governing and Yang Linking Vessels
  -Point of the Window of Heaven, Sun Si-miao Ghost Point
- DU 23 (*shàng xīng*) Upper Star
- DU 26 (*shuǐ gōu*) Water Trough
  -Meeting Point of the Governing Vessel with the Large Intestine and Stomach Channels

To enhance the effect of the selected ghost points, distal points can also be used. When the disturbing dreams and memories are associated with pathogenic heat, the following points are effective for conducting internal heat downward.

Select LV 3 (*tài chōng*), KI 3 (*tài xǐ*), KI 6 (*zhào hǎi*), BL 62 (*shēn mài*), SI 3 (*hòu xǐ*).

Li Dong-yuan's Yin Fire Theory & PTSD Acupuncture

Li Dong-yuan's yin fire theory describes yin fire as a pathological fire that tends to rise upward from the middle and lower burners to harass the upper burner. However, since the heart is a yin viscus with no affinity for yang fire, very often yang fire will attack the small intestine channel, the heart's paired yang channel. Yang pathogens tend to rise upward and affect the head and the neck region. Thus, due to constant worry and thought, the heart will become damaged causing the small intestine channel to also become damaged. In these cases, there will be pain in the scapular region.

Li Dong-yuan also stated that heat in the heart may also affect the *Chong* channel. Since the *Chong* channel is yin in nature and with no affinity for yang fire, yang fire may transfer to the *Du* channel. Since the *Du* channel is yang in nature, yang fire will counterflow upward along the governing vessel and then overflow to the foot and hand *Taiyang* channels, also causing symptoms in all three yang channels.

It is not uncommon for PTSD patients to describe psychological complaints and symptoms associated with the *Du* channel, the heart channel, the small intestine channel, and the urinary bladder channel. Common PTSD symptoms include irritability, depression, profuse dreams, insomnia, neck and shoulder tension and pain, headaches, allergic rhinitis, TMJ, low back pain and weakness, heart palpitations, a feeling of heaviness in the chest, and being easily startled.

Points that can be utilized to treat PTSD symptoms based upon the yin fire theory include:

RN 17 (*dàn zhōng*) (Heart palpitations, chest oppression)

BL 47 (*hún mén*) (Nightmares)

BL 42 (*pò hù*) (Nightmares)

HT 7 (*shén mén*) (Heart palpitations, insomnia)

PC 6 (*nèi guān*) (Heart palpitations)

HT 6 (*yīn xì*) (Fright palpitations)

KI 3 (*tài xī*) (Insomnia, profuse dreams, impaired memory)

KI 6 (*zhào hǎi*) (Nightmares, insomnia)

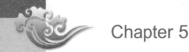

BL 19 (*dǎn shù*) (Irritability, insomnia)

BL 18 (*gān shù*) (Anger)

BL 15 (*xīn shù*) (Impaired memory, heart palpitations)

BL 23 (*shèn shù*) (Lower back pain and weakness)

BL 43 (*gāo huāng*) (Heart palpitations, insomnia)

SI 3 (*hòu xī*) (Back pain)

DU 14 (*dà zhuī*) (Headaches)

GB 20 (*fēng chí*) (Headaches)

Auricular Acupuncture—NADA Protocol

The **NADA** protocol is used extensively by acupuncturists who work with a non-profit organization called Acupuncturists Without Borders. Volunteer acupuncturists are assembled together whenever there is a traumatic public event or natural disaster. Recent examples include their work with first responders at September 11 attacks in New York City, and also the many people affected by Hurricane Katrina.

PTSD is a complex disorder, and effective treatment requires a multi-modality approach to truly enable patients to heal and recover. It should be noted that the **NADA** protocol is recommended to be used in conjunction with standard mental health care.

The **NADA** protocol model can be defined and summarized as follows:

- Clinicians use five ear acupuncture points including ear points Sympathetic, Liver, Kidney, Lung, and *Shenmen*.
- Treatment is provided in a group setting for 40-45 minutes.
- Acupuncture treatment is integrated with conventional elements of psycho-social rehabilitation.

  The Psycho-social Characteristics of the **NADA** protocol:
- It is a non-verbal process: the treatment will be just as helpful even when the patient is reluctant to speak about certain issues.
- The patient can become engaged in therapy even before they are comfortable with intense one-on-one interactions.

- Patients who are trauma victims will be able to participate in treatment even though they remain fearful of interpersonal relationships.
- Acupuncture helps to promote a meditation-like state: patients become comfortable with their own physical processes as a result.
- Acupuncture treatment in a group setting creates an environment that is both reassuring and validating.
- Patients can be treated before assessment and diagnosis are completed so that the patient can remain calm and cooperative enough for a useful diagnosis to be made.
- Developing trust between the therapist and patient becomes easier.
- The patient can relax more easily without losing control.

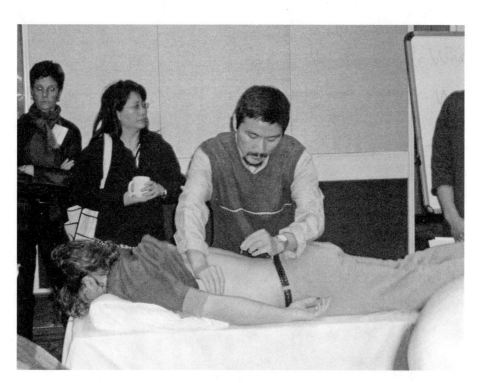

Joe Chang teaching at the AOMA conference, 2009

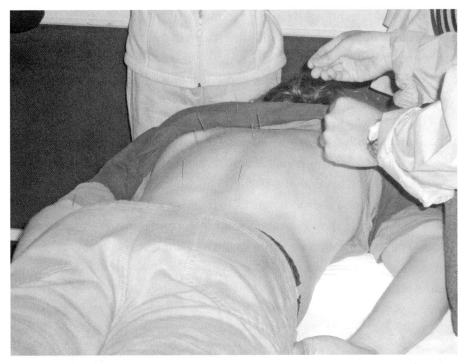

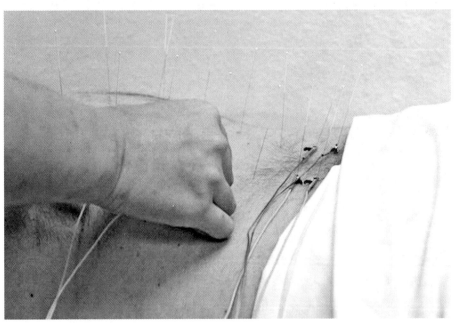

Treating an American soldier with Electro-acupuncture

Chapter 6
Case Studies

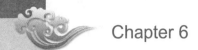

The following case studies are examples of PTSD treatment as provided for veterans of the Iraq and Afghanistan conflicts, and also for victims of the recent earthquake in China's Sichuan Province.

In China, most of the earthquake victims were treated during the acute phase of PTSD, and also in an ER setting. Therefore, the treatment plan was relatively short, with Chinese medicinals and qi-gong therapy as the principal treatment methods.

In the U.S.A., treatment was provided in an outpatient setting for longer periods of time, since many veterans were suffering with chronic PTSD symptoms. A number of patients were treated for up to one year with a variety of integrative treatment methods.

Case Studies from the U.S.A.

CASE STUDY #1

Background Information: 35 year-old male reported a depressed mood and poor attitude for 4 months. He described many exposures to traumatic events starting with the Oklahoma City federal building bombings, 9/11 Twin Towers, Hurricane Katrina, and also combat in Iraq.

Psychological Symptoms: Recurrent, persistent thoughts and images of traumatic events, attempts to avoid and suppress thoughts and images, obsessive behaviors to rid self of guilt and anxiety, recurrent distressing nightmares, avoidance of situations reminding him of the events, feelings of detachment, sleep disturbance, irritability and anger, hypervigilance, and an exaggerated startle response.

General Appearance: Acute distress, but well oriented to time, place, and person.

Current Medications: Prazosin, Hydroxyzine, Zolpidem, Citalopram, Sumatriptin, Promethazine.

【1st Acupuncture Treatment】—June 10, 2008

Subjective: Left hand numbness starting from the scapula and ending at the index and middle finger. Neck pain, with difficulty turning his head. Pain scale: 3/10. Reports anxiety, depression, hyperarousal, and insomnia. After treatment there was reduced hand numbness and the neck showed full range of motion.

Objective: Behaviors demonstrated psychomotor agitation, frustration, anxiety, and anger. Affect was full-ranging, irritable, and agitated; affect congruent with mood. Thought content revealed no impairment. Left hand numbness traveled through the heart channel.

Pulse/Tongue: (L) - wiry, rapid (R) - wiry, rapid. Red tongue with a thin white coating, red at the tip extending through the upper-half of the tongue.

TCM Diagnosis: PTSD with heart-spirit disturbance and liver depression.

Points: Standard acupuncture treatment protocol with added points HT 3 (*shào hǎi*), SJ 5 (*wài guān*), LI 11 (*qū chí*), *bā xié* (EX-UE9); HT 1 (*jí quán*) and HT 3 (*shào hǎi*) for left hand numbness, and one *ashi* point for neck pain.

【5ᵗʰ Acupuncture Treatment】— June 24, 2008

Subjective: Migraines at a pain scale of 7/10, originating at the base of the neck and referring to the temples; also with photosensitivity to light. Anxiety, agitation, and anger improved, also reports lessened depression. Patient fell asleep, and left the treatment with no migraine, less anxiety, and less photosensitivity.

Objective: Frustration, anxiety, and anger improved. Thought content revealed no impairment.

Pulse/Tongue: (L) - wiry, rapid (R) - wiry, rapid. Red tongue with a thin white coating, red at the tip, extending to the upper half of the tongue.

TCM Diagnosis: PTSD with heart-spirit disturbance and liver depression.

Points: Standard acupuncture treatment protocol with added points GB 20 (*fēng chí*), BL 2 (*cuán zhú*), GB 14 (*yáng bái*), *yú yāo* (EX-HN4), *tài yáng* (EX-HN5), and one *ashi* point for neck pain.

【8ᵗʰ Acupuncture Treatment】—July 21, 2008

Subjective: No migraines for three weeks, sleep quality improved. No left arm numbness or pain in the heart channel. Panic attacks and anxiety are much better, but nightmares are persistent. Depression continues to improve. Left shoulder and trapezius pain with neck rotation, pain scale 3/10. Patient left treatment without pain and less anger and anxiety.

Objective: Frustration, anxiety, and anger outbursts have improved. Thought content revealed no impairment.

Pulse/Tongue: (L) - wiry, rapid (R) - wiry, rapid. Red tongue with a thin white coating, red at the tip, extending to the upper-half of the tongue.

TCM Diagnosis: PTSD with heart-spirit disturbance and liver depression.

Points: Standard acupuncture treatment protocol with three added *ashi* points for left shoulder pain.

【Summary】

This PTSD case involved a patient that had been involved in four traumatic events: the Oklahoma City Federal Building bombings, 9/11 Twin Towers, Hurricane Katrina, and combat exposure in Iraq. Subjective symptoms included depression, anxiety, insomnia, recurrent nightmares, and an exaggerated startle response. In speaking with his primary psychologist, the patient seemed to be compartmentalizing the four previous traumas; this is a normal response for someone who has experienced multiple traumatic events.

Because the majority of symptoms pointed to heart and liver channel dysfunction, the main TCM diagnosis was heart-*shen* disturbance and liver depression; however, the enduring nature of the condition also began to affect the kidney. The pulse was wiry and rapid, and the tongue was red with a thin white coating. The tongue was also red at the tip, extending to the upper half of the tongue.

The standard acupoint protocol used in the treatment included LI 4 (*hé gǔ*), SP 6 (*sān yīn jiāo*), ST 36 (*zú sān lǐ*), LV 2 (*xíng jiān*),HT 3 (*shào hǎi*), *yìn táng* (EX-HN3), *Anmian*, DU 20 (*bǎi huì*), KI 3 (*tài xī*), KI 6 (*zhào hǎi*), GB 21 (*jiān jǐng*), BL 15 (*xīn shù*), BL 18 (*gān shù*), BL 20 (*pí shù*), BL 21 (*wèi shù*), BL 23 (*shèn shù*).

Ear tacks were also applied to auricular points Kidney, Heart, Liver.

In Chinese Medicine, there is no separation of the body and mind because the body is viewed as the material basis of the mind. The psyche and physical functions are inseparable and thus can be treated together as in this case. Treating the affected channels with acupuncture benefits the *shen* while also relieving the somatic symptoms (in this case, neck pain and lower back pain). In this case, the treatment principle was to balance the heart and liver channels while also employing spleen and stomach earth points to ground and center the patient.

CASE STUDY #2

Background Information: 30 year-old male reported that one month previously he was in a light armored vehicle that was hit by an anti-tank mine. He denies a loss of consciousness but reports being dazed and confused for a few minutes. He was later evaluated at the aid station. About a week later he was sent to the clinic because of "shaking vision". He was put on a 4-week profile, and medical evacuated. He reports daily headaches and nausea that wax and wane, and at their worst he rates them at 10/10. Has also has difficulty remembering names as well as things he and his wife have done in the past. His concentration level is decreased, he stutters frequently, and his physical balance is impaired. Also reports mood swings and occasional insomnia.

Psychological Symptoms: Recurrent persistent thoughts and images of traumatic events, attempts to avoid and suppress thoughts and images, obsessive behaviors to rid self of guilt and anxiety, recurrent distressing nightmares, avoidance of situations reminding him of the events, feelings of detachment, sleep disturbance, irritability and anger, hypervigilance, and an exaggerated startle response.

Neurological: Speech was abnormal some slow word-finding. Cranial nerves: normal. Motor: a motor exam demonstrated no dysfunction. Cerebellum: no cerebellum coordination-related abnormalities were noted. Balance: normal. Gait and Stance: normal to slightly wobbly tandem gait.

General Appearance: Awake, alert, well oriented to time, place, and person. Well developed, well nourished and hydrated, healthy appearing with no acute distress.

Current Medications: Elavil, Prilosec, Phenergan, Percocet, Seroquel, Sertraline.

【1st Acupuncture Treatment】 — January 15, 2009

Subjective: Post-concussion syndrome headaches located throughout the entire head area, described as a throbbing, aching pain lasting 30-45 minutes with a frequency of once per day. Pain scale average 6-8/10, highest level at 8-9/10 once per week. Other symptoms include photophobia, phonophobia, and nausea, but he denies vision changes and vomiting, jaw claudication, neck/shoulder pain, and scalp tenderness. Patient also reports high anxiety, easy to angry, and a dislike of public places.

Objective: Behavior demonstrated psychomotor agitation; mood displayed frustration, anxious, and anger. Affect was full-ranging, irritable, and agitated; affect was congruent with mood. Thought content revealed no impairment. Observed as physically normal, but with a slightly wobbly tandem gait.

Pulse/Tongue: Pulse was wiry and rapid; the tongue had a white and yellow coating and a red tip.

TCM Diagnosis: PTSD and post-concussion syndrome headaches with heart-spirit disturbance and liver fire.

Points: Standard acupuncture treatment protocol with added *ashi* points for post-concussion syndrome headaches.

【4ᵗʰ Acupuncture Treatment】 — January 27, 2009

Subjective: Pain scale averaged 4/10, never reaching 10/10. Anxiety levels were low, and the patient felt the treatment effect as lasting for three days. No panic attacks reported.

Objective: Behavior demonstrated less agitation, anger, and anxiety. Affect was congruent with mood, and thought content revealed no impairment. Appearance normal, but with a slightly wobbly tandem gait.

Pulse/Tongue: Pulse was wiry and rapid; the tongue had a red tip with a white and yellow coating.

TCM Diagnosis: PTSD and post-concussion syndrome headaches with heart-spirit disturbance and liver fire.

Points: Standard acupuncture treatment protocol with added *ashi* points for post-concussion syndrome headaches.

【8ᵗʰ Acupuncture Treatment】 — February 5, 2009

Subjective: Pain scale averaged of 2/10, never reaching 10/10. Anxiety levels were low, and the patient felt the treatment effect as lasting for three days. No panic attacks reported.

Objective: Behavior demonstrated less agitation, anger, and anxiety. Affect was congruent with mood, and thought content revealed no impairment. Appearance normal, but with a slightly wobbly tandem gait.

Pulse/Tongue: Pulse was wiry and rapid; the tongue had a red tip with a white and yellow coating.

TCM Diagnosis: PTSD and post-concussion syndrome headaches with heart-spirit disturbance and liver fire.

Points: Standard acupuncture treatment protocol with added *ashi* points for post-concussion syndrome headaches.

【12th Acupuncture Treatment】 — February 19, 2009

Subjective: Pain scale averaged 0/10, occasionally reaching 2/10. Anxiety levels were low throughout the week. No panic attacks.

Objective: Behavior demonstrated less agitation, anger, and anxiety. Affect was congruent with mood. Thought content revealed no impairment. Appearance normal, but with a slightly wobbly tandem gait.

Pulse/Tongue: Pulse wiry and rapid; the tongue had a white and yellow coating with a red tip.

TCM Diagnosis: PTSD and post-concussion syndrome headaches with heart-spirit disturbance and liver fire.

Points: Standard acupuncture treatment protocol with added *ashi* points for post-concussion syndrome headaches.

【Case Summary】

This case involved a PTSD patient with a concurrent diagnosis of post-concussion syndrome (mild traumatic brain injury, or TBI). He displayed symptoms of anger, anxiety, a loss of balance, headaches (mostly involving the gallbladder channel), insomnia, poor memory, and depression. The pulse was wiry and rapid, and the tongue was red at the tip with a white and yellow coating.

These signs and symptoms reflect liver/gallbladder channel dysfunction and heart-fire. The standard protocol included acupoints GB 8 (*shuài gŭ*), *yìn táng* (EX-HN3), DU 20 (*băi huì*), GB 20 (*fēng chí*), LV 2 (*xíng jiān*), LI 4 (*hé gŭ*), LI 11 (*qū chí*), BL 15 (*xīn shù*), BL 18 (*gān shù*), BL 19 (*dăn shù*), BL 23 (*shèn shù*).

The focus of treatment was to first address the irritability, depression, post-concussion headaches, and anxiety. The patient seemed to display increased anger and irritability when his anxiety levels were high, and vice versa. In my opinion, this shows a correlation between the liver, gallbladder, and heart channels. From a five phase standpoint, the liver phase feeds the fire phase, so in this case the treatment principle of "sedating the son" was employed. I often needle LV 2 (*xíng jiān*) for patients with signs of liver fire rising (anger, irritability, GB channel headaches) when accompanied by heart-related signs of agitation, anxiety, and disturbed sleep. For GB channel headaches select GB 8, which is in most cases also an *ashi* point. For anxiety, select *yìn táng* (EX-HN3), BL 15

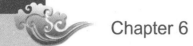

(*xīn shù*), and LI 4 (*hé gǔ*). For memory problems, select DU 20 (*bǎi huì*) and BL 23 (*shèn shù*).

CASE STUDY #3

Background Information: 29 year-old male reported combat stress symptoms including hypervigilance—scanning environments including public places and roadways, increased startle reflex, and flashbacks. He stated that some smells and sounds cause him feel that he is back in Iraq, and feeling somewhat disoriented when he realizes he is back in the USA, c/o feelings of detachment, recurrent and intrusive thoughts of combat experiences, sleep fluctuations, and depression rates at a 6—8/10 at this time. Patient also reported being near multiple IED blasts while in Iraq and stated that he had experienced a brief loss of consciousness, feeling dazed and confused afterwards. He also stated feelings of anger and irritability with difficulty concentrating, memory loss and forgetfulness, also feeling discouraged, helpless and hopeless. He reported financial worries, marital problems, fatigue, hot flashes, decreased libido, loneliness, decreased appetite, difficulty working, and feelings of guilt. Patient also demonstrated psychomotor restlessness.

Psychological Symptoms: Recurrent, persistent thoughts, and images of traumatic events, attempts to avoid and suppress thoughts and images, obsessive behaviors to rid self of guilt and anxiety, recurrent distressing nightmares, avoidance of situations reminding him of events, feelings of detachment, sleep disturbance, irritability and anger, hypervigilance, and exaggerated startle response.

General Appearance: In acute distress, but well-oriented to time, place, and person. Patient did not appear to be experiencing any major discomfort.

Current Medications: Paroxetine, Naproxen, Topiramate, and Midrin.

【Group Psychotherapy】 — March 20, 2009

Subjective: The patient had just attended a combat stress-management group, with continued discussion and processing of chronic post traumatic symptoms. Today's topic was anxiety management, with a discussion on symptoms and coping skills, where he began to verbalize more and open up about his character and how he is changing. He was pleased to report that the acupuncture treatments were helping to release and reduce his "pent up energy", helping him become increasingly free to let go of anger and repressed issues. He was also providing more spontaneous feedback to other group members without solicitation, admitting that as his self esteem continued to increase, his appearance had also become more important. He reported persistent nervousness, but with less frequency and intensity. The group addressed how to specifically deal with past events that are creating maladaptive patterns of behaviors such as avoidance, frustration, isolation, low energy, and poor motivation.

Objective: Patient presented as appropriately groomed, with greater cooperative participation in group discussion. Speech, volume and rate: within normal limits (WNL) for his condition. Mood: verbal, with increased irritability and sadness when reminiscing over the loss of battle colleagues and a family member. Anxiety is noted with concern, affect congruent. Thought processes, thought content, judgment and insight WNL.

【1ˢᵗ Acupuncture Treatment】— March 6, 2009
Chief Complaint

Patient reported high anxiety levels, constant movement of his arms and legs, an inability to relax, insomnia, and an inability to tolerate crowded areas (i.e., Wal-Mart). Reports lower back pain at the L5/S1 level, with migraine headaches located on the right side of the frontal area, above the eyebrows.

History of Present Illness

Problem list reviewed with patient and medication list reviewed with patient. The visit was deployment-related.

Past Medical/Surgical History

Medical: previous psychiatric treatment.

Physical trauma: trauma to the right side of the head.

Diagnosis: head injury.

Personal History

Habits: lack of adequate sleep and frequent changing sleeping positions.

Functional status: self-reliant in normal daily activities.

Subjective

When treated for severe anxiety in a prone position with acupuncture needles placed in the upper and mid-back with electrical stimulation, the

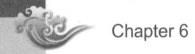

patient reported no discomfort and fell asleep during the treatment.

Review of Systems

Psychological symptoms: continuous anxiety for a month or more.

Physical Findings

Vital signs:

Pain level (0-10) - current lower back pain level 4/10.

General appearance: healthy appearance, awake and alert, well-oriented to time, place, and person.

Treatment Plan

Continue with current therapies.

Discussion

Patient goals: decrease lower back pain to 2/10 within 4 weeks.

【3rd Acupuncture Treatment】— March 20, 2009

Chief Complaint

Anxiety and hyperarousal symptoms of PTSD. After the last treatment, anxiety levels and hyperarousal symptoms were reduced; he also no longer suffered panic attacks when re-experiencing his trauma. Patient felt that acupuncture treatments helped with his PTSD symptoms a great deal as compared to standard mental health treatment.

Subjective

Needles were placed in the upper and lower back for hyperarousal symptoms of PTSD. Patient was treated for one hour with electrical stimulation.

Review of Systems

Psychological symptoms: anxiety.

Physical Findings

General appearance: healthy, alert and active, well-oriented to time, place, and person.

Counseling/Education

Anticipatory guidance: informed that acupuncture may lead to an increased or decreased energy state for the remainder of the day, with euphoric or depressed feelings and possible difficulty sleeping for a night. There may be localized pain at the needle insertion sites.

【Case Summary】

This case is especially interesting because of the specific acupoints that were selected to improve the patient's memory, depression, and psychomotor restlessness. The subjective symptoms of memory loss, insomnia, anxiety, depression, dream disturbed sleep, and lumbago reflect a disconnection of the heart and kidney channels, and the frequent mood swings and angry outbursts point to liver channel involvement. The pulse was wiry and rapid, and the tongue was dry with a white coating and a red tip.

The patient displayed a great deal of psychomotor discharge, anxiety, and hyperarousal symptoms of PTSD. He was constantly moving about and tapping his right leg, as if he was bouncing an infant on his lap, and he was unable to sit still for long periods of time. Therefore, treatment mainly focused on relieving the symptoms of PTSD and traumatic brain injury. After the third treatment, the patient reported that he was able to consolidate all aspects of his traumatic event and could finally recall the time, location, and the sequence of the event.

The psychomotor discharges were associated with a pattern of liver wind, so several liver/gallbladder points were selected: GB 21 (*jiān jǐng*), LV 2 (*xíng jiān*), BL 18 (*gān shù*), and ear point Liver.

For other PTSD symptoms, earth points ST 36 (*zú sān lǐ*) and SP 6 (*sān yīn jiāo*) were used to ground and center the patient.

For anxiety and hyperarousal, ear points Heart, Liver, and *Shenmen* were combined with UB15.

Symptoms of TBI often include memory deficits, depression, and mood changes that include mood swings and angry outbursts. To address these symptoms, the following points were selected: DU 20 (*bǎi huì*) (memory and TBI), *sì shén cōng* (EX-HN1) (memory and TBI), *yìn táng* (EX-HN3) (depression, anxiety, anger), LI 4 (*hé gǔ*) (TBI), KI 3 (*tài xī*) (memory).

The entire acupuncture protocol included points DU 20 (*bǎi huì*), *sì shén cōng* (EX-HN1), *yìn táng* (EX-HN3), KI 3 (*tài xī*), SP 6 (*sān yīn jiāo*), ST 36 (*zú sān lǐ*), LV 2 (*xíng jiān*), BL 15 (*xīn shù*), BL 18 (*gān shù*), BL 23 (*shèn shù*), GB 21 (*jiān jǐng*). Ear tacks were used on both sides at points Heart, Liver, and *Shenmen*.

GULF WAR SYNDROME (GWS) AND PTSD

There is an overlap of symptoms with Gulf War Syndrome (GWS) and PTSD. In both cases, there are symptoms of depression and anxiety followed by physical pain. With PTSD, there may be predominant somatic

pain related to the anxiety, whereas in GWS patients, the pain is usually chronic; most frequently associated with fibromyalgia. GWS patients also most often experience chronic fatigue.

As in the following case, the symptoms of concurrent PTSD and GWS often include chronic fatigue, anxiety, depression, hyperarousal, fibromyalgia, anger, irritability, and migraines. Although medication, psychotherapy, and biofeedback techniques gave some relief, by following an intensive treatment plan including frequent acupuncture, the patient was able to decrease his pain medications by 50%. His quality of life improved as he began to increase his physical activity, and the hyperarousal symptoms, anxiety, anger, nausea, and migraines all decreased dramatically after acupuncture treatment was included.

PATIENT: Male, age 38.

March 28, 2009

Signs and Symptoms: Fibromyalgia pain is constant, level 4/10. Cold rainy days and also poor sleep quality tend to increase his pain levels. Patient reports that his anger, anxiety, and hyperarousal symptoms have improved, but also recently increased stress levels.

History of Present Illness: Problem list reviewed with patient and medication list reviewed. The visit was deployment-related.

Assessment: The patient suffers with a combination of chronic pain symptoms as associated with GWS (migraines, fibromyalgia, nausea, fatigue). He also reports struggling to maintain a positive approach to the confusing aspects of his body's reactions; it seems that he has begun to compensate for the cognitive difficulties and pain in mostly positive ways. PTSD symptoms of anger, anxiety, and depression have improved over time.

Personal History: Habits—Lack of adequate sleep.

Functional status: Physical disability affecting his work, but self-reliant in typical daily activities.

<u>**Review of Systems**</u>

Neurological: Dizziness upon standing up.

Psychological: Signs of both depression and anxiety at moderately elevated levels, problems with affect instability involving anger, high levels of resentment, verbal aggressiveness and aggressive attitudes, with a moderately high level potential for acting-out physical violence.

Physical Findings

General Appearance: Normal appearance, affect congruent with mood. Well oriented to time, place, and person.

Vital Signs: Current (0-10) pain level at 4/10.

Musculoskeletal: General/bilateral tenderness was elicited. Trigger points found positive at the occipital muscles, supraspinatus muscles, and trapezius.

Current Medications: Bupropion, Sertraline, Esomeprazole Magnesium Trihydrate, Tramadol, Fluticasone Propionate (Flovent), Loratadine.

Acupuncture Treatment: DU 20 (*bǎi huì*), SP 6 (*sān yīn jiāo*), ST 36 (*zú sān lǐ*), SP 9 (*yīn líng quán*), *yìn táng* (EX-HN3), GB 8 (*shuài gǔ*). BL 15 (*xīn shù*), BL 16 (*dū shù*), BL 18 (*gān shù*), BL 20 (*pí shù*), BL 23 (*shèn shù*) treated for one hour with electrical stimulation. Moving cupping applied to BL channel.

Treatment Plan: Continue with current therapies. Recommend reduced physical activity, contact sports and high impact activities prohibited.

Discussion

Patient goals: Decrease pain levels to 2/10 within 4 weeks.

Anticipatory guidance: Acupuncture may lead to an increased or decreased energy state for the remainder of the day with euphoria or a depressed feeling. Sleep may be improved or difficult for the first night. Localized pain may appear at the needle insertion sites.

April 20, 2009

Signs and Symptoms: Patient reports less fatigue, migraines, and overall body pain since beginning acupuncture. However, the patient reports recently increased lower back soreness. Anger and irritability has improved with each treatment. Anxiety and hyperarousal has also decreased, with no panic attacks reported.

Acupuncture Treatment: DU 20 (*bǎi huì*), SP 6 (*sān yīn jiāo*), ST 36 (*zú sān lǐ*), SP 9 (*yīn líng quán*), *yìn táng* (EX-HN3), GB 8 (*shuài gǔ*). BL 15 (*xīn shù*), BL 16 (*dū shù*), BL 18 (*gān shù*), BL 20 (*pí shù*), BL 23 (*shèn shù*) treated for one hour with electrical stimulation. Moving cupping applied to BL channel.

Treatment Plan: Continue with current therapies and reduced

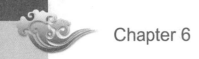

physical activity.

May 8, 2009

Signs and Symptoms: Pain levels were markedly decreased. Hyperarousal levels have decreased as well.

Physical findings

Vital signs: Pain level 5/10.

Musculoskeletal:

General/bilateral tenderness was elicited. Trigger points found positive at the occipital muscles, supraspinatus muscles, and trapezius.

Treatment Plan

Continue with current therapies and reduced physical activity.

Discussion

Patient goals: Decrease pain levels to 3/10 within 4 weeks.

June 11, 2009

Signs and Symptoms: Overall body pain decreased to 2/10. Anxiety levels have decreased. Patient also stated that he has taken nearly 50% less pain medication since beginning acupuncture treatments. Sleep and anxiety both have improved. Patient intends to continue with the current treatment plan.

SUMMARY

In Chinese Medicine, all treatment should follow proper syndrome differentiation. In this case, the symptoms of Gulf War Syndrome manifested as deficiency of the spleen with damp-heat. The patient was fatigued, felt heaviness throughout his body, and had problems with digestion and diarrhea caused by dairy products and uncooked vegetables. His tongue had a thick white yellow coating, and the pulse was slippery and rapid.

The PTSD symptoms manifested mainly as liver qi stagnation, with frequent bouts of anger, irritability, and depression. However, when the flow of liver qi is impaired, the heart may also become disquieted. When this occurred, manifestations also included hyperarousal, anxiety, and insomnia.

Following every acupuncture treatment, moving cupping was utilized following the diagram below. The cup is moved first vertically down the left side of the BL channel from BL 13 (*fèi shù*) to BL 25 (*dà cháng shù*) then horizontally across from the left side of the BL channel to the right side of the BL channel at BL 25 (*dà cháng shù*). The cup is then moved upward from BL 25 (*dà cháng shù*) to BL 13 (*fèi shù*) and then back across to the left side of the BL channel. This method helped eliminate the qi stagnation and discomfort associated with fibromyalgia.

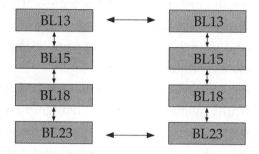

Additionally, the patient was instructed to self-massage specific acupoints for certain conditions. For nausea, the patient was instructed to massage PC 6 (*nèi guān*). For migraines, the patient was instructed to massage GB 8 (*shuài gǔ*). Not only does this increase the therapeutic effect of treatment, but it also empowers the patient, enabling him to self-treat the many symptoms of chronic fatigue, nausea, migraines, anxiety, etc.

It should be noted that for PTSD and GWS, in order to maintain a lasting therapeutic effect, the course of treatment should be long enough, with at least two treatments per week for at least three months. The patient in this case had received over 30 regular acupuncture treatments.

Case Studies from China

CASE 1

April 2006.

Background: 22 year old female, student.

One year previously the patient was involved in a major car accident that was nearly fatal.

Family: She was born in a rural area with 3 siblings. Her parents and elder sister were farmers and they paid for her study expenditures. Her family lived a frugal life and in poor living conditions; because of this, she cherished her educational opportunity and was very dedicated

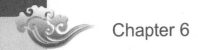

to her studies.

Psychological Symptoms: Since the event, she exhibited an unstable mood with repeated, disturbing memories. She stated that she dislikes crowded areas and would avoid walking outside, especially on the sidewalks. She could not concentrate during classes and had lost all interest in learning; her academic performance had declined as a result. She had frequent nightmares and was often sleepless at night.

General Condition: Clear consciousness, good growth and development, nervous and tearful during the intake, gaunt complexion, she appeared to be both fatigued and hyper-alert.

Four Diagnostic Methods: Poor mood and easily distracted, fatigued, poor memory, difficulty falling asleep, frequent nightmares, poor appetite, and an emaciated appearance. She reported decreased menstruation during the past year, with light-colored menses and a regular cycle. Her complexion and tongue were pale with a thin white and slightly greasy coating. Her pulse was deep, thready, and weak.

Status Analysis: Before the event her mental condition was normal. Afterward her mood was unstable, nervous, and fearful, with intrusive thoughts. She had insomnia, a hyper-alert state, and would avoid school. Up until this visit, she would cry whenever mentioning this event. These symptoms had persisted for more than a year.

TCM Analysis: The heart governs the spirit and the spleen governs thinking. Over-thinking gives rise to consumption of spleen qi and blood with splenic dysfunction leading to poor nourishment of the heart-spirit. Spleen and heart deficiency causes the heart-spirit to lack nourishment, thus the mind cannot remain calm. Manifestations of spleen and heart deficiency include poor mood, poor concentration, poor memory, and insomnia. Spleen deficiency and dysfunction of splenic transportation give rise to internal retention of damp turbidity which manifests with poor appetite, emaciation, and a greasy tongue coating. Spleen and heart deficiency impacts the production of qi and blood which will manifest with the following symptoms: fatigue due to malnourishment of the four limbs; deep, thready and weak pulses; and decreased menstrual flow with pale menses due to poor nourishment of the uterus. Pale complexion and tongue appear also due to malnourishment.

TCM Diagnosis: Spleen and heart deficiency, insufficiency of qi and blood.

Treatment Plan: Introduce procedures → relaxation techniques → regulate sleep → understand the patient's condition clearly → face the trauma → advocate patient interaction in the treatment plan → regain health.

【**First Treatment**】

April 21st 2006

Status: Accompanied by her friends, she held her friend's left hand tightly. She demanded someone to turn the light on and to close the window and door to the room. Her muscles were stiff from after sitting on the chair. She couldn't describe her illness history initially and so supplementary information was provided from her friends. The interview was often disrupted due to her crying. When the event was mentioned, her body shook uncontrollably as tears filled her eyes.

Procedures: Informed consent—first introduce the concept of trauma and traumatic stress responses, the necessity of treatment, and any possible problems and prognosis as related to treatment. Obtain verbal consent for voluntary participation and also to cooperate with her primary physician throughout the treatment.

Breathing and Relaxation Techniques: While seated, perform self-relaxation treatment through regulation of the breath.

Chinese Medicinal Formula:

Guī Pí Tāng (Spleen-Restoring Decoction)

人参	*rén shēn*	15g	Radix Ginseng Alba	
白术	*bái zhú*	15g	Rhizoma Atractylodis Macrocephalae	
茯苓	*fú líng*	30g	Poria	
黄芪	*huáng qí*	20g	Radix Astragali	
龙眼肉	*lóng yǎn ròu*	15g	Arillus Longan	
酸枣仁	*suān zǎo rén*	30g	Semen Ziziphi Spinosae	Baked
当归	*dāng guī*	15g	Rhizoma et Radix Araliae Cordatae	
木香	*mù xiāng*	15g	Radix Inulae	
远志	*yuǎn zhì*	10g	Radix Lysimachiae Insignis	Prepared

continued

炙甘草	*zhì gān cǎo*	6g	Radix et Rhizoma Glycyrrhizae Praeparata cum Melle	Prepared
龙骨	*lóng gǔ*	30g	Os Draconis	Calcined
郁金	*yù jīn*	20g	Radix Curcumae	
谷芽	*gǔ yá*	20g	Fructus Setariae Germinatus	Baked
麦芽	*mài yá*	20g	Fructus Hordei Germinatus	Baked

Formula Analysis:

This formula contains *Sì Jūn Zǐ Tāng* (Four Gentlemen Decoction), containing *rén shēn* (Radix Ginseng Alba), *bái zhú* (Rhizoma Atractylodis Macrocephalae), *fú líng* (Poria), *zhì gān cǎo* (Radix et Rhizoma Glycyrrhizae Praeparata cum Melle), and also *huáng qí* (Radix Astragali), all of which act together to strengthen the spleen and tonify qi.

Suān zǎo rén (Semen Ziziphi Spinosae) and *dāng guī* (Rhizoma et Radix Araliae Cordatae) nourish blood and calm the spirit, *yuǎn zhì* (Radix Lysimachiae Insignis) with *suān zǎo rén* (Semen Ziziphi Spinosae) and *lóng gǔ* (Os Draconis) tranquilize the mind and promote sleep, and *mù xiāng* (Radix Inulae) and *yuǎn zhì* (Radix Lysimachiae Insignis) act to resolve dampness.

Yù jīn (Radix Curcumae) relieves depression and dissipate masses; *gǔ yá* (Fructus Setariae Germinatus) and *mài yá* (Fructus Hordei Germinatus) invigorate the spleen and harmonize the stomach.

This formula combination acts to tonify the heart and spleen and replenish qi and blood to treat the root. It can also tranquilize the mind, regulate the mood and promote sleep to address the main manifestations.

Analysis:

The patient showed symptoms of hyperarousal characterized by an inability to concentrate and difficulty falling asleep. Symptoms of avoidance included an unwillingness to talk about the traumatic event and avoiding situations that reminded her of the trauma.

Treatment here should focus mainly on relaxation training in order to relieve the anxiety and improve sleep quality. The treatment plan also includes a Chinese medicinal formula combined with standard mental health protocols and music therapy. Cognitive behavior therapy is applied to reduce symptoms of hyperarousal and avoidance behavior.

【2nd Treatment】

April 27th

Status: The patient arrived by herself, without request of turning on the light, and sat on the chair voluntarily. With an apathetic expression, she described clearly her feelings, but during the interview she would lower her head, or play with the ornaments on her clothes. She didn't mention the traumatic event, but repeatedly emphasized that she wanted to change her current status and that she wanted her life back. During her descriptions, she said that she wanted to cry, but that she was able to control her mood.

Treatment Procedures

➢ **Music and Relaxation Therapy:** The patient lies down while listening to soft music, calming the mind gradually for about 30 minutes with a combination of relaxation and breathing exercises.

➢ **Cognitive Behavioral Therapy:** Teach the patient smile consciously, promote self-satisfaction and self-praise, utilize examples from daily life. Suggest a goal or task in order create a concrete reason for self-praise.

➢ **Environmental Therapy:** Suggest visiting public parks with her friends near the school.

➢ **Chinese Medicinals:** After taking the decoction, her appetite improved and nightmares were reduced. 4 to 6 more decoctions of the same formula were prescribed.

➢ **Exercise:** Continue the 24-style tai-chi form for 20 to 30 minutes before bedtime.

Analysis: Arriving unaccompanied to the clinic showed that confidence had been successfully established between the patient and doctor. However, hyperarousal symptoms remained very high, and she avoided speaking about the traumatic event directly. Treatment continued to focus on relaxation training in order to calm the mind and reduce anxiety. Environmental suggestions were given to help her spend the upcoming holiday safely in a natural environment that promotes self-healing, while Tai-chi practice would help to improve her mental focus.

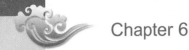

Chinese medicinals and tai-chi both can help to improve sleep quality.

【3rd Treatment】

May 12th

Status: Patient arrived by herself, and smiled when she entered the room. She immediately reported that she could fall asleep easier, and that she felt more relaxed and less agitated.

Treatment Procedures:

➢ **Music Therapy:** With soft music playing, inquired as to how she spent time during the holiday.

➢ **Relaxation Therapy and Suggestion:** Patient was asked to lie on the treatment table for three-line relaxation practice. When relaxed, she was treated with suggestion therapy to help her face past events. The procedure lasted for about 40 minutes.

➢ **Emotional Guidance Therapy:** Discuss the clinical manifestations of acute distress, talking freely with the patient about the traumatic event, including the impact on her studies, daily life, and social activities. This method aims at helping the patient go through the process by inducing the emotion, describing the emotion, and understanding the emotion. Questions asked during therapy included:

1. What was your most painful problem after the traumatic event?

2. What are your disturbing thoughts and memories? What are the triggers that are inducing anxiety?

3. Which negative beliefs or values have resulted from the event? Or, what beliefs have been changed by the event? How have they changed?

After this discussion, help the patient to reconstruct the negative beliefs and to develop new coping mechanisms.

Treatment lasted for 20 minutes. The patient would stop communication occasionally, without crying, but with deep breathing and sighing.

➢ **Exercise:** Regular tai-chi practice.

➢ **Chinese Medicinals:** Because the patient's menstrual period was approaching, *jī xuè téng* (Caulis Spatholobi) and *shān zhā* (Fructus Crataegi) were added to the formula, and *yuǎn zhì* (Radix Lysimachiae Insignis), *gǔ yá* (Fructus Setariae Germinatus) and *mài yá* (Fructus Hordei Germinatus) were removed.

3 daily decoctions were prescribed, to be withdrawn during menstruation.

Analysis:

Improvement in her sleep quality indicated greater stability in mood; voluntary smiling shows that a good connection had been established between the patient and the doctor. Emotional guidance therapy was used gradually to help her face the traumatic event more directly.

Since the greasy tongue coating was now absent, *yuǎn zhì* (Radix Lysimachiae Insignis) was removed; because menstruation was approaching, *jī xuè téng* (Caulis Spatholobi) was added to nourish and activate the blood. *Shān zhā* (Fructus Crataegi) replaced *gǔ yá* (Fructus Setariae Germinatus) and *mài yá* (Fructus Hordei Germinatus) to strengthen the spleen, harmonize the stomach, activate blood, and regulate menstruation.

【4th Treatment】

May 17th

Status: The patient seemed to be in a good mood, having brought a CD of her favorite music. When describing the entire traumatic event as requested, she appeared to maintain a stable mood.

Treatment Procedures

➤ **Catharsis Therapy:** When describing the event, she confirmed that she felt depressed, so she was asked to sing along with her favorite song as loudly as possible.

➤ **Adaptation Therapy:** Breath regulation and eye movement desensitization was applied while allowing the patient to recall the traumatic event. When recalling the anxiety-arousing stimulus, massage was applied along with acupressure to points [*shén mén* (HT 7), *nèi guān* (PC 6), *zú sān lǐ* (ST 36), *sān yīn jiāo* (SP 6)]. Adaption therapy enables the patient to adapt and eventually remove all of the physical and motor discharges associated with the trauma (palpitations, muscular bracing of the shoulders and the back, clenched fists and jaws). The anxiety-arousing stimuli were induced in combination with music therapy, lasting for 30 to 40 minutes each time, for 3 weeks in total.

➤ **Chinese Medicinals:** Menstruation arrived on May 16th with increased flow and normal color. Sleep quality was good, with no

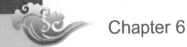

nightmares for 2 weeks, so patent medicinals were prescribed.

Xiāo Yáo Wán (Free Wanderer Pills) and *Guī Pí Wán* (Spleen-Restoring Pills), 6g TID.

【5th/6th Treatments】

May 19th / 26th

Treatment procedures were similar to the 4th treatment, but a greater variety of anxiety-arousing stimuli were induced. She was also encouraged to communicate more frequently with her friends.

Analysis: During the third treatment, the patient could face the trauma more directly. The frequency of treatment was increased to consolidate the therapeutic effect by scheduling the 4th treatment four days later, and a 5th treatment two days after that.

【7th Treatments】

June 2nd 2006

Status: The patient reported feeling much better, stating that she was now able to focus on her studies and prepare for her final exams. She was communicating freely with her classmates, no longer avoided public areas, and was again able to drive. No panic attacks or depression had appeared since she began driving.

Treatment Procedures

➢ **Music Therapy:** The patient enjoyed her own music, independently regulating the volume.

➢ **Breath Regulation:** Breathing exercises were practiced, and she was advised to self-regulate her breathing whenever nervous or under stress.

➢ **Cognitive Therapy:** Reminded her to continue smiling consciously, and to also practice self-praise.

➢ **Chinese Medicinals:** Patent formulas *Xiāo Yáo Wán* (Free Wanderer Pills) and *Guī Pí Wán* (Spleen-Restoring Pills) were continued in between menstrual periods.

Discussion: Therapist and patient had comprehensive discussion of the content, experience, gains, and remaining issues of treatment, focusing on the clinical effect and the positive impact that had been gained.

Analysis: The patient had improved greatly, and felt that she could finally continue with her life. However, three-step relaxation practice and other techniques (i.e., music therapy, environment therapy, tai-chi, and breathing exercises) should be continued.

CASE 2

Background: A 13-year-old boy was brought to the clinic by his uncle. One month previously when returning from school, he found his parents dead and lying on the floor of their home. Since then he had become an orphan.

Psychological Symptoms: Indifferent, depressed, and unfocused.

General Condition: Conscious and well-nourished.

Four Diagnostic Methods: Depressed mood, normal appetite, and regular urination and bowel moments. Red tongue with a thin yellow coating, and a wiry pulse.

Status Analysis: Before the traumatic event, he was an easygoing boy with healthy relationships, but after the event he became extremely sad and withdrawn with a predominantly apathetic expression. There was also some acting out of hostility and anger toward the surrounding environment. All of these symptoms had been present for the entire month.

Syndrome Analysis: The heart governs the spirit, and sudden fear and sorrow leads to poor nourishment of the heart, manifesting here with apathy and insomnia. Liver qi stagnation also gives rise to a depressive mood. The red tongue with a yellow coating and wiry pulses suggest liver qi stagnation with poor nourishment of the heart.

Intervention Procedures: Counseling was given to help the patient release his sorrow and depression. The patient was taught to self-regulate his emotions, also verbally encouraged through language guidance and suggestion. Cognitive behavioral therapy was employed to correct his misconceptions of the traumatic event.

【1st Treatment】

October 15th 2007

Impression: Patient felt sad and cried bitterly. He could control his emotion when the event was mentioned; however there were some fluctuations which indicated suppressed feelings.

Treatment: With 3-line relaxation training, patient was asked to recall the traumatic event with language guidance therapy, and then encouraged to release his repressed emotions. He was then counseled and encouraged to foster a positive attitude in daily life.

【2nd Treatment】

October 17th

Impression: He seemed to feel better and said that he felt like crying, but could not. His depressed mood had improved, but he did not want to discuss the traumatic event.

Treatment: Continue the same treatment plan with 3-line relaxation therapy and emotions and desire techniques. Suggestion techniques and language guidance was applied to encourage him to continue his studies. At the end of treatment, he had regained a normal mental status.

Analysis

The abnormal status of this patient was caused by a traumatic event, and only psychological therapies and relaxation methods were required. Since the patient was suppressing fear and sadness, counseling methods were used to help enable him to release negative emotions. The patient was later encouraged with suggestion and language guidance methods.

CASE 3

【1st Treatment】

June 19th 2008

Background: A 14-year-old female student, grade 6. On May 12th 2008, she had sustained a head injury during the Sichuan earthquake. Both of her parents were immigrant workers, so she had been staying with her grandmother who had also become injured. The patient had been normally cheerful until after the event occurred.

Psychological Symptoms: Extremely fearful, avoided talking about the earthquake, lonely, easily distracted, unable to concentrate on her entrance exam for middle school, tossing and turning during sleep, often waking. She seemed to be full of bitterness, but also trying to look happy so that others would not worry.

General Condition: Conscious and well-nourished, a sad expression, and a 10 cm scar on her head.

Four Diagnostic Methods: Nervous, anxious, unable to speak about the traumatic event, becomes extremely fearful when she mentions the traumatic event, poor sleep and waking often. Normal appetite, urination, and bowel movements. Hypomenorrhea with dark menses.

The tongue was red with thin yellow coating and ecchymosis, and her pulse was rough.

Status Analysis: Before the earthquake, she had a lively and cheerful personality with normal social relationships. Afterwards, she was often nervous and fearful and was reluctant to talk about the traumatic event. She was hypervigilant, also displaying avoidance behaviors that impacted her normal daily life and studies. When mentioning the event her mood would change and she would become depressed and extremely fearful. All symptoms lasted for one month, thus meeting the diagnostic criteria of PTSD.

TCM Analysis: The heart governs the spirit, and sudden suffering or fear and fright leads to poor nourishment of the heart-spirit, manifesting here with a depressed mood. The liver is considered as the basis of menstruation, and it also stores the *hun*, or ethereal soul. Yin deficiency of the heart and liver leads to the liver failing to control the *hun*, resulting in poor sleep. Deficient heart qi fails to promote blood circulation, and the liver governs the free flow of qi. Qi stagnation also leads to poor blood circulation, manifesting with hypomenorrhea and dark colored menses, ecchymosis on the tongue, and a rough pulse. In summary, the syndrome here involves yin deficiency of the heart and liver with disturbance of the heart-spirit.

Intervention Procedures: Counseling to help release repressed emotion, and teach the patient to self-regulate her mood, and cognitive behavioral therapy to correct misconceptions of the traumatic event.

Chinese Medicinals: To tonify yin and calm the spirit, modified *Tiān Wáng Bǔ Xīn Dān* (Celestial Emperor Heart-Supplementing Elixir) was prescribed.

【2nd Treatment】
June 20th 2008

Impression: The patient reported feeling better since the last treatment, and also that she was not so frightened of the earthquake. Although her parents didn't stay together with her, her aunt's family members were very friendly towards her, and her grandmother would return soon from Nanjing. She was now staying with her elder sister in a campsite, where she would often write in her diary.

Treatment: Counseling to help with repressed emotion, followed

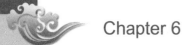

by instruction in breathing and relaxation exercises. She was advised her to practice these exercises whenever she was in a poor mood, and encouraged to communicate more with her classmates and teachers.

Analysis

The abnormal status of this patient was caused by a traumatic event, and the patient suppressed her sadness and grief. Treatment began with counseling, followed by self-help techniques for regulating mood and fostering a positive attitude.

CASE 4

Background: A 13-year-old female student, grade 6. On May 12th 2008 when the earthquake occurred, she barely escaped the classroom. The classroom collapsed killing three students and one teacher. Several hours later, her father was also injured in the earthquake.

Psychological Status: Depression, sadness and a desire to cry; she also felt that it was very unfair that her father was hurt. She was angry and very irritable.

General Condition: Well-developed and well-nourished, with a sad expression.

Four Diagnostic Methods: Low mood, easily distracted, fatigue, frequent nightmares, normal appetite, regular urination and bowel movements. The tongue was red with a yellow coating, her pulse was slippery.

Status Analysis: Before the earthquake, she had a cheerful personality with normal social relationships. After the earthquake she was sad, angry, irritable, and experienced frequent nightmares. She was reluctant to recall the traumatic event, also displaying symptoms of avoidance which affected her daily life and studies. All of these symptoms had persisted for one month.

TCM Analysis: The heart governs the spirit, and fear and fright leads to poor nourishment of the heart-spirit causing frequent nightmares. The liver governs the free flow of qi, and depressed emotions give rise to qi stagnation which transforms into fire. The red tongue with a yellow coating and slippery pulses also indicate hyperactivity of liver and heart fire with disturbance of the heart-spirit.

Intervention Procedures: Counseling to help release repressed emotion while also instructing the patient to self-regulate her mood. Cognitive behavioral therapy is then applied to correct misconceptions of the traumatic event.

Chinese Medicinals: Modified *Dān Zhī Xiāo Yáo Sǎn* (Free Wanderer Powder plus Cortex Moutan and Fructus Gardeniae) and *Dǎo Chì Sǎn* (Red Guiding Powder).

Exercise: Morning practice of *Ba Duan Jin* dynamic qi-gong for one hour on the reconstructed playground.

【1ˢᵗ Treatment】

June 19ᵗʰ, 2008

Impression: Depressed mood, unable to control her crying, also anxious and worried about her father's injury.

Treatment: Her mood was stabilized her mood with breath regulation, and when relaxed, cognitive therapy helped her to understand that natural disasters are unavoidable and that everyone will have fear, and that injury cannot be avoided. She was encouraged to express and her emotions verbally and through journal writing.

【2ⁿᵈ Treatment】

June 20ᵗʰ, 2008

Impression: She reported an improved mood since the last treatment; also her father's condition had become less serious. Her attitude was more positive in that she believed that all of her family members and neighbors would continue to help each other. She felt less alone, and had begun to interact again with her younger sister. During treatment, her mood was stable.

Analysis:

The abnormal status of this patient was caused by a traumatic event, and she was clearly suppressing sadness. She was taught to release her depression and self-regulate her mood. Cognitive therapy was used to correct her misconceptions that her father's injury could have been avoided; she was also encouraged to communicate with her family members and foster a positive attitude.

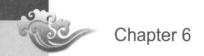

CASE 5

Background: a 45 year old male from the hardest-hit disaster area in Sichuan Province, where his son had lost his life in the earthquake. He waited for three entire days at the gate of the school, finally carrying his son's body out of the ruins by himself.

Psychological Symptoms: Hyperarousal, irritability, vexation, aggression, difficulty falling asleep.

General Condition: Conscious and well-nourished.

Four Diagnostic Methods: Hyperarousal, irritability, vexation, difficulty falling asleep, and aggressive behavior. Red tongue with thick yellow coating, and a rapid slippery pulse.

Status Analysis: The patient was an easygoing person before the earthquake, but had become extremely sad due to the loss of his son. The other manifestations of hyperarousal, irritability, and aggressive behavior towards others also had affected his daily life. All symptoms had persisted for one month, thus meeting the diagnostic criteria of PTSD.

TCM Analysis: The heart governs the spirit, where sudden suffering and fear leads to poor nourishment of heart-spirit and difficulty falling asleep. Hyperactivity of liver fire manifests with irritability and vexation. Tongue and pulse signs also indicate hyperactivity heart and liver fire with disturbance of the heart-spirit.

Exercise: Morning practice of *Ba Duan Jin* dynamic qigong for one hour on the reconstructed playground.

Intervention Procedures: Counseling to help release repressed emotion, instruct patient to self-regulate his mood. Cognitive behavioral therapy is then applied to correct misconceptions of the traumatic event.

Chinese Medicinals: To clear liver fire and calm the spirit, Modified *Chái Hú Jiā Lóng Gǔ Mǔ Lì Tāng* (Bupleurum Decoction Plus Dragon Bone and Oyster Shell) and *Dǎo Chì Sǎn* (Red Guiding Powder) was prescribed.

【1st Treatment】

June 8th, 2008

Impression: Hyperarousal, anger, irritability, and difficulty falling asleep (4 tablets estazolam were ineffective). He initially refused treatment, even shouting at the doctors.

Treatment: Counseling was given to help him release repressed emotion. The patient was visited by counselors every evening as well. The following three interventions employed the same methods.

【5th Treatment】

June 12th, 2008

Impression: Vexation and unstable emotions; he missed his son very much. However, he was now able to talk with his therapists without displaying hostility.

Treatment: Counseling, language guidance therapy, instructed to practice breath regulation exercises each day.

Analysis:

The abnormal status of this patient was caused by the loss of his son, causing both excitation and anger. Because it was difficult for him to accept the truth, he attributed his son's death to the outside world; he was irritable and initially refused treatment from a psychologist. For the initial stage of treatment, listening with conviction was most essential. Counseling methods were effective in helping him deal with his repressed emotion; finally, breathing and relaxation self-help methods were provided.

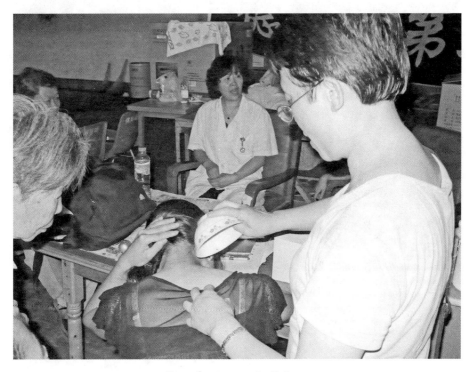

Gua-sha therapy in Sichuan

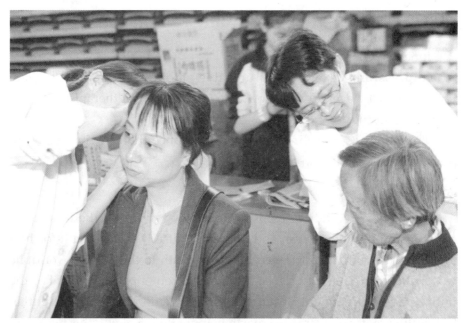

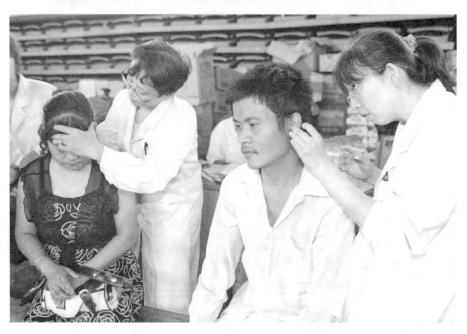

Auricular therapy in the Sichuan clinic

Chapter 7
Current Research on
PTSD Treatment

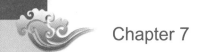

To date, research on the effects of Traditional Chinese Medicine (TCM) in the treatment of post-traumatic stress disorder (PTSD) in China has been limited due to the relative lack of subjects afflicted with this disorder. However, with the recent earthquake in Northern China, some new research and case studies have appeared. Western studies have also been published concerning increased serum cortisol, growth hormone levels, and immune cytokine disturbances in those Northern Chinese earthquake survivors with PTSD.

However, a number of Chinese studies have been recently published on the effects of TCM on depression, anxiety, and generalized anxiety disorder (GAD). Depression and anxiety often severely impact patients who are diagnosed with PTSD. These studies can shed some light on various TCM approaches, where the treatment of depression and anxiety are a significant part of the treatment approaches for PTSD patients.

TCM Research on PTSD

In Li Zhong-yi and He Rui-fang's study[1], 62 PTSD patients were randomly divided into a treatment group and a control group. The treatment group received amitriptyline (100–150 mg/d) along with a combination of a Chinese medicinal decoction (1 decoction/day) to reduce side effects. The control group received Western pharmacotherapy consisting of amitriptyline only.

Functioning to enrich yin and calm the mind, the prescribed decoction contained *dì huáng* (Radix Rehmanniae) 18g, *tiān dōng* (Radix Asparagi) 15g, *mài dōng* (Radix Ophiopogonis) 15g, *mǔ dān pí* (Cortex Moutan) 18g, *dì gǔ pí* (Cortex Lycii) 24g, *shí hú* (Caulis Dendrobii) 15g, *běi shā shēn* (Radix Glehniae) 18g, *suān zǎo rén* (Semen Ziziphi Spinosae) 9g, *tiān huā fěn* (Radix Trichosanthis) 15g, *tǔ yuǎn zhì* (Radix Lysimachiae Insignis) 15g, *shí chāng pú* (Rhizoma Acori Tatarinowii) 15g, *gǒu qǐ zǐ* (Fructus Lycii) 9g, *nán wǔ wèi zǐ* (Fructus Schisandrae Sphenantherae) 9g, *chuān xiōng* (Rhizoma Chuanxiong) 6g, *fú shén* (Sclerotium Poriae Pararadicis) 5g, *tǔ dāng guī* (Rhizoma et Radix Araliae Cordatae) 10g, and *dān shēn* (Radix et Rhizoma Salviae Miltiorrhizae) 9g.

Dà huáng (Radix et Rhizoma Rhei) (decocted last) and *zhǐ shí* (Fructus Aurantii Immaturus) were added for severe constipation; *màn jīng zǐ*

(Fructus Viticis), *bái jí lí* (Fructus Tribuli), and *gōu téng* (Ramulus Uncariae Cum Uncis) were added for severe headache.

In the control group, amitriptyline (100–150 mg/d) was given over a course of 12 weeks, and low dosages of non-benzodiazepines such as chloral hydrate and zolpidem were applied in those patients with insomnia.

Evaluation was performed before the treatments, 6 weeks after treatments and 12 weeks after treatment, including the Hamilton Anxiety Scale (HAMA), Zung Self-Rating Depression Scale (SDS), and Traumatic Exposure Severity Scale (TESS).

There were no significant differences in curative effect and score-reducing rates, but the response time of the subjects in the integrative Western and Chinese Medicine treatment group experienced quicker therapeutic effects and fewer side effects as compared to the control group.

Studies on Northern Chinese Earthquake Survivors

There are two current Western studies conducted at Beijing University on Northern Chinese Earthquake Survivors with PTSD. In one study, researchers found a correlation of increased serum cortisol and growth hormone levels (GH) in those earthquake survivors with PTSD. The 30 earthquake survivors diagnosed according to the DSM-IV criteria displayed significantly elevated serum cortisol levels and higher GH levels as compared to the control group. This research further supports the growing body of evidence that the pathology of PTSD involves a component of the neuroendocrine system.

The second research suggests the involvement of immune cytokines in the pathophysiology of PTSD patients. In this study, serum interleukin (IL)-2, IL-6 and IL-8 levels were compared between earthquake survivors with PTSD, those with non-PTSD, and normal controls. In a 3-armed study, 34 earthquake survivors with PTSD (according to DSM-IV criteria), 30 earthquake survivors with non-PTSD, and 34 controls were recruited in northern China using the Composite International Diagnostic Interview instrument. Researchers concluded that the earthquake survivors diagnosed

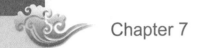
with PTSD had a significant correlation with lower serum IL-8 levels. Additionally, the severity of depression and anxiety symptoms was positively related to serum IL-6 levels.

TCM Research on Depression and Anxiety

In an article published in *Journal of Sichuan Traditional Chinese Medicine* (#1, 2001, p. 27-28) titled "40 Cases of Phlegm Fire Pattern Generalized Anxiety Disorder Treated with *Qīng Xīn Dí Tán Tāng* (Clear the Heart & Flush Phlegm Decoction)" researchers designed a study involving a treatment intervention group and a control group. The cohort was comprised of 77 patients with a mean age of 30 ± 5.7 years and a mean disease duration of 11 ± 5.78 years. There was no significant statistical difference between these two groups ($P < 0.05$) in terms of their age, sex, or disease duration.

All of the subjects were diagnosed with generalized anxiety disorder. Additionally, the subjects underwent a battery of tests that involved a pre/post treatment examination that included blood analysis, urine analysis, liver and kidney function, ECG, as well as the Hamilton Anxiety subjective distress rating scale.

The treatment group was given the Chinese medicinal formula *Qīng Xīn Dí Tán Tāng* (Clear the Heart & Flush Phlegm Decoction): *huáng lián* (Rhizoma Coptidis), *chái hú* (Radix Bupleuri), *zhī zǐ* (Fructus Gardeniae), and *dǎn nán xīng* (Arisaema cum Bile), 15g each; *huáng qín* (Radix Scutellariae), *shí chāng pú* (Rhizoma Acori Tatarinowii), and *suān zǎo rén* (Semen Ziziphi Spinosae), 20g each; *yuǎn zhì* (Radix Polygalae) 10g, and *cí shí* (Magnetitum) 30g.

One packet of these medicinals was decocted in water per day and administered in three divided doses. The comparison group received Valium 1mg TID.

The researchers concluded that the study resulted in a total effectiveness rate of 80% for the treatment intervention group and 83.8% in the comparison group. Analysis of the clinical outcomes suggests statistically significant changes in both the treatment group as well as the comparison group, with the treatment group recording fewer side effects as compared with the comparison group.

In another study conducted at the Changshu Municipal Chinese Medical Hospital in Changshu, Jiangsu province and is titled "The Treatment of 38 Cases of Anxiety Disorder with *Huáng Lián Wēn Dǎn Tāng* (Coptis Warm the Gallbladder Decoction)", researchers designed a study involving a treatment intervention group and a control group. The cohort comprised of 38 patients with a Chinese medical pattern differentiation diagnostic pattern of phlegm heat with internal exuberance.

Treatment consisted of the herbal formula *Huáng Lián Wēn Dǎn Tāng* (Coptis Warm the Gallbladder Decoction): *huáng lián* (Rhizoma Coptidis), 6g, *zhú rú* (Caulis Bambusae in Taenia), 12g, *zhǐ qiào* (Fructus Aurantii), 12g, *bàn xià* (Rhizoma Pinelliae), 6g, *fú líng* (Poria), 12g, and *chén pí* (Pericarpium Citri Reticulatae), 6g.

One packet of these medicinals was decocted in water and administered in three divided doses per day. The researchers concluded that the study resulted in a total effectiveness rate of 84%.

In another study titled "Observations on the Therapeutic Efficacy of Treating 176 Cases of Psychological Depression by the Methods of Acupuncture for Regulating the Liver" researchers designed a 3-armed study at conducted at several different hospitals and provinces in China from October 2004 to December 2006.

The cohort comprised of 440 subjects diagnosed with unipolar depression according to the Hamilton Depression Rating Scale (HAMD) and who also exhibited either the pattern of liver qi depression or qi depression transforming into fire. The 440 subjects were randomly assigned to three groups: 1) a liver-regulating acupuncture treatment group, 2) a Prozac treatment group, and 3) a sham acupuncture group.

In the liver-regulating acupuncture group, there were 176 subjects, in the Prozac treatment group 176 subjects, and in the sham acupuncture group 88 subjects. In terms of age, sex, and disease duration, the three groups were considered statistically comparable for the purposes of this study.

All members of the liver-regulating acupuncture group were needled at the following acupoints:

Si Guan: The Four Bars, LV 3 (*tài chōng*), and LI 4 (*hé gǔ*)

DU 20 (*bǎi huì*)

Yìn táng (EX-HN3)

LV 3 (*tài chōng*) and LI 4 (*hé gǔ*) were needled perpendicularly to a depth of 0.5 *cun*. Needles were manipulated until the *deqi* sensation was obtained, and then retained for 30 minutes. In addition, auricular acupuncture using press needles was applied unilaterally at the Liver and Heart earpoints. These needles were retained for three days and then switched to the opposite ear. This treatment was carried out two times per week for a total of three months.

All members of the sham acupuncture group were needled at points different than the liver-regulating acupuncture group. Needles were manipulated until the *deqi* sensation was obtained, then retained for 30 minutes. In addition, auricular acupuncture using press needles were applied at different auricular points as compared to the acupuncture intervention group. These needles were retained for three days and then switched to the opposite ear. Treatment was carried out two times per week for a total of three months.

All members of the Prozac treatment group were orally administered 20mg of Prozac per day for three months.

The researchers concluded that at the end of the three month follow-up, the liver-regulating acupuncture group as a whole experienced a significantly better reduction in their HAMD scores than did the Prozac group or the sham acupuncture group. The sham acupuncture group resulted as the least effective method as compared with the Prozac group and the liver-regulating acupuncture group.

In another study, Yang Yong-cheng and Xie Dao-jun published an article in *Henan Traditional Chinese Medicine* (#6, 2000, p. 36-37) titled, "A Clinical Audit of 36 Cases of Depression Treated by Combined Chinese & Western Medicines." The researchers designed a study comparing the outcomes of one group of patients treated only with Western psychiatric pharmacotherapy and another group which received concurrent Chinese and Western medical treatments.

The cohort consisted of 36 patients in the treatment group who received concurrent Chinese and Western medical treatments, and 22 patients were treated with Western pharmacotherapy alone in the comparison group. All the patients in this study were diagnosed with unipolar depression according to the criteria published in Chinese National Criteria for the Differentiation & Diagnosis of Psychiatric Diseases, 2nd edition, also referred to as the CCMD-2. There were no significant statistical differences between the members of these two groups in terms of age, sex, disease course, or hospital status.

The comparison group received either 150-250mg of amitriptyline per day, 150-200mg of clomipramine, and/or two tablets of Dai An Shen (Indigo Spirit-quieter; a common Chinese brand sedative).

The treatment group also received modified *Xiāo Yáo Sǎn* (Rambling Powder): *chái hú* (Radix Bupleuri), 15g, stir-fried *bái zhú* (Rhizoma Atractylodis Macrocephalae), *bái sháo* (Radix Paeoniae Alba), *dāng guī* (Radix Angelicae Sinensis), and *fú líng* (Poria), 10g each, and *bò hé* (Herba Menthae) and *gān cǎo* (Radix et Rhizoma Glycyrrhizae), 6g each.

The outcomes of this study were assessed using the Hamilton Rating Scale for depression. In the comparison group (received only Western pharmacotherapy) the total effectiveness rate in this group was 77.3%. In the treatment group which received both Chinese medicinal and Western pharmacotherapy, the total effectiveness rate in this group was 88.9%. There was a marked statistical difference in the outcomes between these two groups (P < 0.05).

PTSD Research in the United States

Currently in the United States there is one study funded by the National Institutes of Health (NIH) on the efficacy of acupuncture in the treatment of Post-Traumatic Stress Disorder. However, because patients diagnosed with PTSD can also have concurrent symptoms of depression, anxiety, and insomnia, studies that have shown the efficacy of acupuncture in the treatment of depression, anxiety, and insomnia are summarized below. Additionally, outcomes measures are summarized on the utilization of the NADA five ear point protocol in the treatment of first responders at Ground Zero for symptoms of anxiety and stress.

The randomized controlled trial by Hollifield et al. (2007) indicated that acupuncture may be efficacious for reducing symptoms of posttraumatic stress disorder (PTSD), depression, anxiety, and impairment in adults diagnosed with DSM-IV-TR PTSD. Adults diagnosed with PTSD were randomized to either acupuncture treatment, group integrated cognitive-behavioral therapy (iCBT), or a wait-list control (WLC). The primary outcome measure was self-reported PTSD symptoms at baseline, end-treatment, and three-month follow-up. Repeated measures MANOVA was used to detect predicted Group X Time effects.

Compared to the WLC condition, acupuncture provided large treatment effects for PTSD (F [1, 46] = 12.60; P < 0.01; Cohen's d = 1.29), similar in magnitude to group iCBT (F [1, 47] = 12.45; P < 0.01; d = 1.42) (ACU vs. iCBT, d = 0.29). The secondary outcomes for depression, anxiety, and impairment in daily functioning were similar to the effects for PTSD, and both treatment groups improved significantly more than the WLC group. The Group X Time contrast from baseline to end treatment was significant for comparing acupuncture versus WLC for depression (d's = 0.83 vs. 0.12, P < 0.01), anxiety (d's = 1.28 vs. 0.19, P < 0.01), and global impairment scores (d's = 0.75 vs. 0.04, P = 0.01). Similarly, CBT versus WLC for depression (d's = 1.08 vs. 0.12, P < 0.01), anxiety (d's = 1.28 vs. 0.19, P < 0.01), and global impairment scores (d's = 0.76 vs. 0.04, P < 0.01). Symptom reductions at end-treatment were maintained at three-month follow-up for both interventions.

Similarly, a study by Spence et al. (2004) indicated that acupuncture might be efficacious for reducing anxiety and insomnia in anxious adult subjects who complained of insomnia.

In the study, 18 anxious adult subjects who complained of insomnia were assessed in an open pre-post clinical trial study. Five weeks of acupuncture treatment was associated with a significant (P = 0.002) nocturnal increase in endogenous melatonin secretion (as measured in urine) and significant improvements in polysomnographic measures of sleep onset latency (P = 0.003), arousal index (P = 0.001), total sleep time (P = 0.001), and sleep efficiency (P = 0.002). Significant reductions in state (P = 0.049) and trait (P = 0.004) anxiety scores were also found. Since this study had significant outcomes in the anxious adult population with insomnia, acupuncture may be effective for the treatment of insomnia and anxiety in post-traumatic stress disorder patients.

The National Acupuncture Detoxification Association (NADA) protocol has been used to treat post-traumatic stress disorder patients, mainly to reduce their stress and anxiety levels. Further evidence for the value of the NADA protocol for the treatment of stress emerged from the 9/11 catastrophe. A Manhattan hospital near Ground Zero set up a trauma relief program immediately after the attack. NADA style acupuncture was included along with Reiki energy work as part of an integrative stress management program.

The St. Vincent's Hospital project gathered data on 99 patients aged 20-83. The first group of subjects received standard NADA 5 ear-point acupuncture alone, and the second group received both ear needling and Reiki treatment. The two groups were very similar in how they rated their stress level pre-treatment on a 0-4 self assessment scale (2.43 and 2.64 respectively).

Following treatment, the groups' average scores improved to 1.33 and .96. Statistical analysis of the scores shows that the improvement by both groups was statistically significant (P < 0.01) but the difference between the groups was not significant.

Gulf War Illness Research in the United States

Research Study—Effectiveness of Acupuncture in Treating Gulf War Illness

The research team at NESA is currently working on a grant funded by the Department of Defense to study the effectiveness of acupuncture in the treatment of Gulf War Illness (GWI). Soon there will be an opportunity to recruit 120 veterans who have this medical diagnosis, and provide them with a robust, individualized, TCM-style acupuncture treatment protocol. As practitioners and scholars of OM, we often look to our tradition's long clinical history of healing patients. However, as was the case with conditions like HIV/AIDS, SARS, and PTSD, new diseases will arise and challenge us to apply TCM as a living model to new clinical problems.

Background

Gulf War Illness (GWI) is a chronic, multi-symptom condition that affects more than one fourth of the nearly 700,000 U.S. military personnel who served in the first Gulf War (1990-91). U.S. and UK troops exhibited the highest prevalence of Gulf War Syndrome as compared to the other nations, possibly due to higher usage of pesticides and anthrax vaccines and higher rates of exposures to oil fire smoke. France troops had the lowest incidence, possibly due to lower usage of pesticides, organophosphate pesticides, and no use of anthrax vaccines. Nineteen years later, many of these men and woman are still affected by symptoms that are sometimes disabling, and no specific treatment has been identified. One case definition of the illness identifies symptom clusters in 3 domains:

- Fatigue that persists 24 hours or more after exertion.
- Pain affecting muscles and joints, with or without known injuries.
- Mood and cognition problems, including feeling depressed, anxious, irritable, or worried, sleep problems, and difficulties with memory and word finding.

As these symptoms suggest, patients given the diagnosis of GWI often have co-morbidities including chronic fatigue syndrome, fibromyalgia, anxiety, and depression. Because we know that many patients with these conditions can be helped by acupuncture, we hope that acupuncture may also prove helpful for GWI.

GWI Case Definition/ CDC

The Centers for Disease Control and Prevention (CDCP) defined CMI complex as the presence for 6 months or longer of one or more self-reported symptoms from at least two clusters of symptoms: Fatigability (Cluster A), Mood and Cognition (Cluster B), and Musculoskeletal Pain (Cluster C).

Each symptom complex was characterized as "mild-moderate" or "severe," for which at least one symptom in each cluster was required to be severe. (Blanchard 2006)

Cluster A: Fatigability	Cluster B: Mood and Cognition	Cluster C: Musculoskeletal
Persistent fatigue 24 hours or more after exertion	Depression	Joint pain or muscle pain
	Irritability	
	Difficulty thinking or concentrating	
	Worry, tension, or anxiety	
	Problems finding words	
	Problems getting to sleep	

Co-Morbidity of PTSD and Gulf War Syndrome

In Gulf War veterans, severe trauma is associated with PTSD and other psychiatric conditions. The federally mandated Research Advisory Committee on Gulf War Veterans' Illnesses released a 452-page report indicating that Gulf War veterans, in addition to displaying symptoms common to Gulf War Syndrome (chronic fatigue, fibromyalgia, depression, etc.), also often have psychological symptoms such as PTSD and anxiety. A majority of the psychological trauma in Gulf War veterans can be attributed to the 18,000 chemical alerts that went off during the Gulf War, accounting for 66% of the psychological trauma. 43% of veterans attribute their psychological trauma to nearby SCUD explosions and 27% of the Gulf War veterans attributed their psychological trauma to combat.

There is also growing evidence to support the co-morbidity of fibromyalgia (one of the major symptoms of Gulf War Syndrome) and psychiatric conditions (PTSD, depression, anxiety). The Research Advisory Committee on Gulf War Veterans' Illnesses report stated that approximately 23% of U.S. and UK troops diagnosed with Gulf War Syndrome have symptoms of fatigue, 18% of U.S. and UK troops have symptoms of muscle and joint pain, 17% have symptoms of migraines, and 32% have impaired cognition. These symptoms are all of common symptoms in fibromyalgia patients.

Approximately 30% of fibromyalgia patients have major depression at the time of diagnosis; the lifetime prevalence of depression is 74% and that of an anxiety disorder is 60%. Additionally, in a study done by Toomey et al. on the mental health of U.S. Gulf War veterans, mood disorders and anxiety disorders such as depression and PTSD were more prevalent in Gulf War veterans that were deployed as compared to veterans that were not deployed. Thus, a link between PTSD and Gulf War Syndrome has been reported, where both conditions share similar symptomatology and pathogenic mechanisms.

Causes of GWI

After many years of study, epidemiologists have recently concluded that symptoms of GWI are most likely due to neurological damage following exposures to neurotoxicants during the war. Severity of

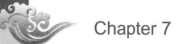

symptoms is highly correlated with two known exposures: use of a medication pyridostigmine bromide (PB), given as a pre-treatment for soman nerve agent poisoning, and use of pesticides.

These substances were used most extensively by ground troops in forward areas on the battlefield and are linked to the most severe cases. Effective protection against weaponized nerve agents does not exist, so US forces were deployed with PB and protective clothing and gear to try to prevent massive casualties. The medication, never before given to healthy subjects, is an acetylcholinesterase inhibitor, metabolized by the liver and excreted by the kidneys, which leads to an excess of the neurotransmitter acetylcholine, an action similar to that of other chemical nerve agents and pesticides to which soldiers were exposed.

Excess cholinergic stimulation of muscarinic receptors of the parasympathetic nervous system results in increased tearing, sweating, salivation, and bronchial secretions, nausea, abdominal cramping and diarrhea. Excess stimulation of nicotinic receptors in the skeletal muscles leads to muscle twitching, cramps, weakness, tremors, and paralysis. CNS effects may include fatigue, mental confusion, poor concentration, and headache. Numerous first person accounts provide details of these side effects experienced by the troops, which subsided after the medication was discontinued or the dosage reduced.

In addition to PB, the second major exposure linked to GWI is pesticides and insecticides, used extensively to protect against the risk of infectious diseases from the numerous insects common to the hot desert environment and unsanitary conditions. Numerous products were applied topically and to uniforms, bedding, and tents. Surveys conducted after the war identified patterns of overuse in forward areas, which have been corrected in subsequent conflicts through changes in product design and usage. PB medication and pesticides are considered as major causes of neurological damage associated with GWI after tracking specific exposures to soldiers with most severe symptoms in a dose/dependent manner.

Among subsets of soldiers, symptoms may be linked to more localized exposures. Some soldiers handled radioactive depleted uranium residues on exploded munitions and equipment during the ground war and its aftermath.

An estimated 100,000 troops were exposed to low level sarin and other toxins when aerosol particles and dust were released into the wind during demolition of chemical weapons stores and interception of Iraqi missiles. Some soldiers report they became ill after extensive refueling of infantry vehicles, or working with de-greasing solvents, or painting vehicles and supplies. The severe desert heat, combat stress, and multiple exposures may have contributed to exacerbated effects of the chemical exposures.

Numerous veterans testified before congressional subcommittees that they first experienced symptoms while in close proximity to such exposures, starting during the air war on January 1991. Many more complaints surfaced within several months of their return home during the fall of that year. These first-person accounts suggest that multiple chemical sensitivities are associated with at least some cases of GWI. There is evidence that a first chemical exposure causes biological changes that increase vulnerability to subsequent exposures, and it is possible that multiple exposures contributed to the most severe cases of GWI.

Stress may be one factor in the etiology of GWI; however, the disease is clearly distinct from the anxiety disorder, PTSD. Stressors associated with deployment and combat are common to all wars, but soldiers are not returning from the current wars in Iraq and Afghanistan with symptoms of GWI. Continued stress associated with struggling with a chronic illness may be a factor in GWI, as the condition was not recognized as service-related until 1998, at which time the military assumed responsibility for medical care and disability benefits.

The acute phase of this disease was largely ignored as soldiers performed their routine duties of war on the battlefield. More than 19 years later, many affected veterans still struggle with debilitating symptoms. The incidence of amyotrophic lateral sclerosis (ALS) in Gulf War veterans is twice that of other groups. The incidence of brain cancer in those affected downwind of the destruction of chemical weapons stores is twice that of other groups. Veterans have also reported birth defects in children conceived soon after returning home, and of symptoms transmitted to family members, perhaps from infectious disease or contaminated clothing and gear.

Meredith St. John, Academic Dean, New England School of Acupuncture
Lisa Conboy, Co-Chair of Research, New England School of Acupuncture

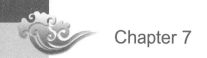

Traumatic Brain Injury (TBI)

As stated in the book titled *Neuropsychology of PTSD*, "A traumatic brain injury (TBI) can be open, resulting from the skull and dura being penetrated by a sharp object (penetrating injury), or closed, resulting from a blow to the head causing a rapid acceleration-deceleration of the brain, or severe rotational forces (as when a car turns over)." The current conflicts in Iraq and Afghanistan involve a greater number closed traumatic brain injury due to increased encounters with improvised explosive devices (IED). Symptoms of TBI can include cognitive deficits, depression, anxiety, irritability, dizziness, light and noise intolerance, headaches, and blurred vision. In the current War on Terror in Iraq and Afghanistan, there were 1,179 TBI medical evacuations during 2006.

Co-Morbidity of PTSD and TBI

A majority of evidence suggests that PTSD can coexist with TBI. In the study by Harvey et al. (2003), titled *Coexistence of Traumatic Brain Injury and Posttraumatic Stress Disorder: Resolving the Paradox*, the researchers stated that "It has been argued that individuals who sustain a TBI and have no conscious memory of their trauma will not experience fear, helplessness and horror during the trauma, nor will they develop re-experiencing symptoms or establish the negative associations that underlie avoidance symptoms. However, single case reports and incidence studies suggest that PTSD can be diagnosed following TBI." Other researches based on case studies have also reached the same conclusion regarding the coexistence of PTSD and TBI with reported rates of PTSD in head-injury victims ranging from 20% to 40%.

Diagnosis and Classification of TBI

Measures of TBI severity include the Glasgow Coma Scale (which is scored by assessing a patient's eye-opening, motor, and verbal responses), length of loss of consciousness, and length of post-traumatic amnesia; about 80 percent of patients with known TBIs are categorized as "mild TBI."

- Two conditions must be met to diagnose a history of TBI:
➤ There must have been an injury event.

> The injury event must have resulted in the person experiencing an alteration of consciousness (ranging from dazed and confused to loss of consciousness).

  • Classification of TBI:

> Mild TBI causes loss of consciousness lasting less than 1 hour or amnesia lasting less than 24 hours.

> Moderate TBI produces loss of consciousness lasting between 1 and 24 hours or post-traumatic amnesia for 1 to 7 days.

> Severe TBI produces a loss of consciousness for more than 24 hours or post-traumatic amnesia for more than 1 week.

Glasgow coma scale		
Eye opening		**Score**
	spontaneously	4
	to speech	3
	to pain	2
	none	1
Verbal response	orientated	5
	confused	4
	inappropriate	3
	incomprehensible	2
	none	1
Motor response	obeys commands	6
	localises to pain	5
	withdraws from pain	4
	flexion to pain	3
	extension to pain	2
	none	1
Maximum score		15

Appendix 1
Implications for Public Health

There is significant relevance in the integration of CAM modalities with standard mental health protocols, especially the integration of acupuncture into military medicine. According to the RAND study[58], the prevalence estimates for PTSD is 5 to 15 percent. If we apply these estimates to the 1.64 million service-members who have already been deployed, we can estimate that the number of individuals returning home with PTSD will range from 75,000 to 225,000.

Projected costs for the treatment of PTSD per person for the two years following deployment ranges from $5,635 to $13,935. Total costs for the treatment of PTSD per person ranges from $422,625,000 to $1,045,125,000 for the estimated 75,000 individuals diagnosed with PTSD. And total costs for the treatment of PTSD per person ranges from $1,267,875,000 to $3,135,375,000 for an estimated 225,000 diagnosed with PTSD.

Given the relative low costs for the use of acupuncture in pain management as illustrated by Spira[59] 2008 (an estimated total cost savings of $128,768.64 for one year of acupuncture treatments as compared to pharmacotherapy), there would be significant cost savings in the treatment of PTSD with acupuncture.

Additionally, the military relevance of employing acupuncturists in military medical centers can be viewed from another economic perspective. In a study conducted by The RAND Corporation[58], researchers estimate that PTSD and depression among returning service members will cost the nation as much as $6.2 billion in the two years following deployment—an amount that includes both direct medical care and costs for lost productivity and suicide. For a typical service person returning from Iraq or Afghanistan (an E-5 with 5 to 7 years of service), a baseline scenario predicts that two-year post-deployment costs will range from $5,635 to $13,935 for PTSD.

Standard mental health therapies include pharmacotherapy and cognitive-behavioral therapy in the treatment of PTSD, and with no significant improvement from standard mental healthcare, the individual would be discharged from the military. This results in the disbursement of life-long veteran benefits that the Congressional Budget Office (CBO) estimates to be between $7 and $9 billion over the period 2008 through 2017 for Afghanistan and Iraq veterans. The RAND Corporation estimates that the government could save as much as $1.7 billion, or $1,063 per returning veteran through evidence-based research; the savings come from increases in productivity, as well as from reductions in the expected number of suicides.

In 2008 the Pentagon spent $5 million on research in seeking new ways to treat troops suffering from combat stress or brain damage by researching alternative methods such as acupuncture, meditation, yoga, and the use of animals in therapy.

Acupuncture is one form of treatment that can help reduce indirect costs and the cost of medical care as evident in pain management. In an article written in 2008 by Commander Spira of the U.S. Navy in Military Medicine, it was stated that the cost savings for one week of outpatient acupuncture therapy for a single patient would be approximately $18.76 per patient. The total cost for one week of pharmacotherapy utilizing Celecoxib is $20.58, as compared to the cost of needles for one week of outpatient acupuncture treatment of $1.82. Additionally, the article stated that 132 different patients were seen at the outpatient acupuncture clinic. Thus, the total estimated cost savings for one week of treatments would be $2,476.32. Acupuncture treatments for pain management as compared to pharmacotherapy for one year would give us a total cost savings of $128,768.64.

Furthermore, in terms of a reduction of indirect costs from outpatient acupuncture therapy, the article states that there was a decrease in sick quarters and light limited duty status resulting in an increase in operational man-days during Operation Iraqi Freedom.[59]

Appendix 2
Post-Traumatic Stress Disorder—Western Perspectives

Combat induced post-traumatic stress disorder (PTSD) is an anxiety disorder diagnosed in 24% of injured active duty combat veterans serving in Iraq and Afghanistan[45]. Onset of PTSD directly relates to multiple and lengthy combat related deployments and trauma[46], with approximately one in six soldiers showing signs of PTSD upon leaving Iraq and Afghanistan. Symptoms of PTSD include re-experiencing, avoidance behaviors, numbing responsivity, hyperarousal, as well as anxiety and insomnia. Unresolved PTSD becomes chronic, and symptoms may continue for life[47].

Several neurotransmitters appear to be closely linked to the etiology of anxiety. PTSD is hypothesized to be a disorder of hyperarousal, which has been supported by research on the autonomic nervous system and hypothalamic-pituitary-adrenal axis function[48]. In patients who have been diagnosed with PTSD, abnormally high levels of catecholamine and cortisol are released during stress. In addition, an increase in sympathetic-adrenal-medullary system activation is common in PTSD patients, which results in an increase in heart rate, blood pressure, startle response, and plasma catecholamine output[49].

The serotoninergic system is also believed to be involved in the regulation of depression. A widely accepted measurement of depression in humans is the measurement of serotonin output through urine analysis, and this pattern is abnormally low in patients who are diagnosed with PTSD. Patients with PTSD have suppressed levels of serotonin and are more likely to have histories of depression as compared with normal patients.

Traditional treatment strategies for PTSD have emphasized selective serotonin reuptake inhibitors that have been shown to reduce symptoms in all three PTSD diagnostic clusters (e.g., intrusion, avoidant/numbing, and hyperarousal). However, the risks of selective serotonin reuptake inhibitors use involve physical as well as psychological effects that include acute toxicity in overdose if they are taken with monoamine oxidase inhibitors or pain-relief medications such as tramadol and sumatriptan[50]. Other side effects of selective serotonin reuptake inhibitor use include sedation, cognitive impairment, agitation, memory loss, and in extreme cases, hallucinations[51].

PTSD Epidemiology

The prevalence of PTSD in the U.S. population is estimated to be between 1 and 12 percent with a higher incidence in at-risk populations such as combat veterans, inner-city children, citizens and refugees of post conflict countries, and victims of terrorist attacks. On average, 25% of individuals experiencing one or more traumas develop PTSD. Symptoms occur in everyone (i.e., 98%). Roughly 80% recover and do not develop PTSD, and about 20% do not recover and develop PTSD. Pre-traumatic risk factors include: history of prior trauma, psychiatric history, and family psychiatric history[55].

PTSD Symptom Clusters

PTSD is an anxiety disorder that develops in response to a traumatic experience and is characterized by the core features of re-experiencing, avoidance behaviors, numbing responsivity, and hyperarousal[51]. Symptoms that characterize the symptom cluster of re-experiencing includes recurrent distressing memories of the event, recurrent dreams of the event, flashback episodes, and bodily reactions to situations that remind them of the traumatic event. Symptoms that characterize the symptom cluster of avoidance include an inability to remember important aspects of the trauma, lack of interest in normal activities, feelings of detachment, a sense of having no future, emotional "numbing", and reduced expression of moods. Symptoms that characterize the symptom cluster of hyperarousal include outbursts of anger, sleeping difficulties, difficulty concentrating, and hypervigilance[51].

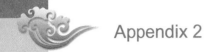

Pathophysiology of PTSD

PTSD affects three main regions of the brain: The amygdala, medial prefrontal cortex, and the hippocampus. The amygdala is a medial temporal lobe structure that appears to be involved in the assessment of threat-related stimuli which also plays a crucial role in the process of fear conditioning. High levels of catecholamine and cortisol release during stress enhance the functioning of the amygdala, promoting fear conditioning. Evidence suggests that the amygdala may be hyper-responsive in individuals with PTSD. The medial prefrontal cortex is the region of the brain that is involved in the extinction of fear conditioning and the retention of extinction. There is an abnormal extinction of fear responses in PTSD. Clinically, PTSD patients experience only minimal declines in fear responses over repeated presentations of traumatic reminders, and the medial prefrontal cortex is hypo-responsive. The hippocampus is involved in memory processing. Severe stressors and high levels of stress-related hormones can be associated with memory impairment and hippocampus cell damage[55].

Neuroendocrine Alterations in PTSD

Neuroendocrine alterations in PTSD involve mainly the hypothalamic-pituitary-adrenal (HPA) axis and the sympathetic-adrenal-medullary (SAM) system. In the sympathetic-adrenal-medullary (SAM) System, an increase in SAM system activation is common in PTSD patients that results in an increase in heart rate, blood pressure, startle response, and an increase in plasma catecholamine output (epinephrine & norepinephrine). Chronic HPA axis over-activation results in low levels of cortisol output, presumably because there is an enhanced negative feedback inhibition[55].

Neurobiology of PTSD

There are several neurobiological dysfunctions in PTSD. Noradrenergic sensitization presumably lies at the basis of hyperarousal symptoms. Opioid dysfunction may underlie some of the numbing symptoms seen in PTSD. Dopamine dysfunction may mediate symptoms of hypervigilance and paranoia. Cortisol mediated damage to the hippocampus may underpin problems in memory. Serotonin depletion may also be a factor in the development of depression and aggression[55].

Neurophysiology of PTSD

The Stress Response

When confronted with extreme stress, the body initiates many chemical reactions to facilitate a quick escape from stress. The amygdala is the brain region that alerts the body to danger and activates hormonal systems. Activation of the hormones noradrenaline and adrenaline result in accelerated breathing, pulse, and heart rate, and an increased release of energy to muscles and other organs which literally helps people run faster from stress or mobilize a response that requires coping with the stressor head-on. Once the immediate danger has passed, other hormones help terminate stress-activated reactions, particularly the hormone cortisol. Usually, the more stress there is, the more cortisol is needed to contain the stress response. Research has demonstrated that trauma survivors with PTSD have higher levels of noradrenaline (Yehuda 1992; Yehuda 1998) and lower levels of the hormone cortisol (Yehuda 1990; Yehuda 1993; Yehuda 1995).

Hormonal Alterations in Trauma Survivors

Trauma survivors tend to experience the world in a state of hyperarousal. Many will display exaggerated physical reactions to normal environmental signals, such as loud noises, and others perceive their environment as a constant threat. They may also display signs of hypervigilance, constantly securing the space around them. According to Dr. Yehuda's research, it appears that "the exaggerated physical reactions to stress in the aftermath of a traumatic event appear to be related to this altered hormonal balance that is in part a result of the traumatic event. It has been particularly interesting that cortisol levels are low in PTSD, since levels of this hormone are elevated in major depressive disorder, a condition that shares many symptoms with PTSD."

A diminished level of cortisol reduces the body's stress response. Low levels of cortisol stress hormones decrease the autonomic nervous system's ability to fully restore itself to a homeostatic state after a traumatic event. Studies have demonstrated that trauma survivors with PTSD exhibit higher levels of noradrenaline (Yehuda 1992; Yehuda 1998),

but lower levels of the hormone cortisol (Yehuda 1990; Yehuda 1993; Yehuda 1995). This may explain the exaggerated startle responses that trauma survivors often display.

Research studies have shown low urinary or plasma cortisol levels in various groups of trauma survivors with PTSD. According to Dr. Yehuda's research, these groups include: Persian Gulf war veterans (Kellner 1997), Vietnam veterans (Yehuda 1990; Yehuda 1993), Korean War and World War II veterans, holocaust survivors (Yehuda 1995), adolescents exposed to earthquake (Goenjian 1996), adult survivors of childhood sexual abuse (Stein 1997), rape victims (Resnick 1995) and motor vehicle accident victims (Yehuda 1998). In contrast, cortisol levels are high in trauma survivors diagnosed with major depression (Yehuda 1990).

Additionally, trauma survivors with PTSD appear to have altered immune system changes. Trauma survivors may have increased rates of illnesses associated with low levels of cortisol. Also, low cortisol levels may be a chemical marker for assessing the trauma survivors' risk of developing PTSD. Low cortisol levels are typically shown in trauma survivors that have developed PTSD.

Biochemistry

Cortisol is a known stress hormone with levels that increase following acute stages of stress, and decrease following relaxation therapies such as massage therapy and acupuncture. Cortisol is an end-product of the sympathetic system. In Dr. Field's research titled, "Cortisol Decreases and Serotonin and Dopamine Increase Following Massage Therapy," cortisol reduction following massage therapy has been noted in conditions ranging from job stress to depression to HIV and breast cancer.

Serotonin is a neurotransmitter that is activated by the central nervous system. Dr. Field's research states that "serotonin is thought to interact with dopamine and cortisol in complex ways, although it can generally be said that serotonin enhances the production of dopamine and hampers the production of cortisol".

Similarly, like serotonin, dopamine is also a central nervous system neurotransmitter. Abnormally low levels of dopamine and serotonin can clinically increase a patient's levels of depression and its stress effects.

Appendix 3

East meets West in a Multidisciplinary Assessment and Treatment Approach for Post-Traumatic Stress Disorder

Marie Sprague, D.O.

Introduction

As a board certified (by the American Board of Psychiatry and Neurology) United States Army psychiatrist for the past seven years I have evaluated and/or treated roughly 9,000 patients with Post Traumatic Stress Disorder (PTSD) triggered by exposure to combat in the wars in Iraq and Afghanistan. I have also assessed and treated civilian populations throughout my career that had their PTSD triggered by car accidents, felony assaults (physical abuse, attempted murder by a sole assailant, robbery), and sex crimes (child molestation, rape, incest), however the main focus of this chapter will be to outline an integrated view of the biology (body), psychology (mind) and energy (spirit) of PTSD related to combat veterans. As a disclaimer, the biological and psychological sections will reference well-established Western resource materials and accepted medical theories and practices, and the energy sections will reference commonly accepted beliefs in Eastern religion/ philosophy, as well as Western authors who have published and lectured on energy medicine in the United States. The views of integrating the three as it relates to PTSD are attributed to my own personal experience and anecdotal evidence, not from specific DOD (Department of Defense) or APA (American Psychiatric Association) guidelines or teachings. It is my understanding that this textbook mainly focuses on Chinese medicinal (herbal, acupuncture and energy meridian) treatment modalities for combat-related PTSD, however a Western psychiatrist's perspective that has some moderate knowledge of energy systems is being included at the end in hopes of providing a more comprehensive understanding of PTSD,

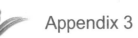

with the end goal of outlining and establishing a successful treatment approach. It has been my experience that when both Eastern and Western approaches are used in a receptive patient in the right context as opposed to a single modality, the potential for sustained remission and improved social and occupational functioning increases by several magnitudes.

PTSD as defined by Western Psychiatry

According to the DSM-IV TR (Diagnostic and Statistical Manual of Mental Disorders, Fourth Edition, Revised) established by the APA, a person must be exposed to a traumatic event in which *both* the actual or threat of death and/or serious injury to self/others *and* his or her emotional response to this traumatic event involved either intense fear, horror, or helplessness in order to meet the first diagnostic criteria that defines PTSD.[1] The latter part of the first criteria (the emotional response of intense fear, horror or helplessness) becomes particularly poignant as it relates to the Eastern view of human energy systems, and in particular to how one Western author (Caroline Myss, Ph.D.) correlates this emotion to human physiology and spiritual development. If a person meets this first criteria, and as a result of witnessing or experiencing this traumatic event he or she reports re-experiencing, increased arousal, and avoidance symptoms that are of clinical relevance for longer than thirty days after the event occurred, then the person fulfills the diagnostic criteria for PTSD. At least one re-experiencing symptom (nightmares, flashbacks [a dissociative episode in which a person "relives" a traumatic experience in the present time], intrusive thoughts of the trauma, psychological distress or physiological reactivity to reminders of the traumatic event), two symptoms of increased arousal (difficulty falling/staying asleep, irritability, hypervigilance, exaggerated startle response, or difficulty concentrating), and three avoidance symptoms (extreme efforts to avoid activities/thoughts/reminders of the trauma, decreased interests in participating in social activities, inability to recall aspects of the trauma [usually due to a dissociative state], feelings of detachment/numbness from others, sense of foreshortened future) must be present in order to meet full diagnostic criteria for PTSD.[1]

The Biology of PTSD

PTSD is the only psychiatric disorder that is defined by etiology, not symptomatology. Anecdotally this has been rephrased in psychiatric academic circles as "PTSD is the only acquired psychiatric illness" because one must experience a trauma in order to meet criteria for the diagnosis. Biological structures and neurochemical dysregulation of the brain have long been theorized to correlate with various psychiatric disorders; PTSD is no exception. Research investigating the biological processes of this illness is gaining momentum as the number of soldiers from various countries exposed to combat who become (and remain) symptomatic increases worldwide. It has been a steadfast psychiatric theory that amygdala and hippocampal dysfunction plays a central role in the pathophysiology of PTSD due to their respective roles for encoding emotion and memory. Simply put, the amygdala encodes the "emotional" component of a memory as the hippocampus simultaneously encodes the "narrative" aspect of a specific experience before the memory is stored in the cortex. In the late 1990's a "split" between the amygdala and hippocampus was theorized to occur in PTSD such that emotional and narrative streams of a traumatic event were stored separately in the medial prefrontal cortex. Shin, Rauch and Pitman[2] did a comprehensive review of the medical literature in 2006 summarizing a decade's worth of neuro-imaging research for PTSD. Their comprehensive review lends some credence to this "split" function theory. They found several studies that support disharmony between these two structures in the formation of traumatic memory in individuals afflicted with PTSD. More specifically, research supported heightened amygdala responsivity during symptomatic states and decreased volume, function, and integrity of the hippocampus, in addition to hyporesponsiveness of the medial prefrontal cortex.[2]

The hypothalamic-pituitary-adrenal (HPA) axis has also been theorized to play a biological role in the pathophysiology of PTSD. A "split" pattern was also seen in several studies that were attempting to assess the role of stress hormones in PTSD subjects. An exaggerated cortisol response was demonstrated in studies designed to stimulate the HPA axis using cognitive cues for traumatic memory, and subjects who were pharmacological challenged with a low dose dexamethasone-

135

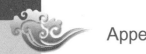
suppression test (DST) showed cortisol suppression.[3] When an individual is stressed, cortisol helps provide energy to the body but usually causes free radical and oxidative damage, triggering the release of glucocorticoids (corticotrophin release factor [CRF]) that are designed to help repair the effects of high-stress states. Cortisol suppresses the sympathetic nervous system and levels are proportional to the magnitude of the stressor. These two hormones are both thought to occur at lower levels in PTSD patient populations, and this is also one theory as to why hippocampal volume decreases (due to cellular damage). Additional studies have also tried to establish if other hormonal differences can be quantified in patients with PTSD, and some observed elevated concentrations of both corticotropin-releasing hormone (CRH)[4], endogenous endorphins[3] (which could psychologically correlate to the "numbing" reported by PTSD sufferers) and norepinephrine.[4]

Also called noradrenalin, norepinephrine serves a dual role as both a stress hormone and a neurotransmitter, is almost identical in composition to epinephrine, and exerts effects on large areas of the brain when released. Noradrenergic neurons originate both in the locus coeruleus (brain stem) and the lateral tegmental field (norepinephrine neuronal tracts), and axons of the neurons in the locus coeruleus act on adrenergic receptors in many areas of the brain, however the structures that are most pertinent to the pathophysiology of PTSD are the neocortex, amygdala and hippocampus. The essence of PTSD is that of CNS autonomic dysfunction in response to trauma, and norepinephrine plays a central role because it is released from postganglionic neurons of the sympathetic nervous system in response to stressful events. It is essentially responsible for transmitting the "fight-or-flight" response. Alertness and arousal are inherent to norepinephrine's biological activity and are also two primitive cognitive states that are dysfunctional in PTSD. Noradrenergic activity was found to be at higher levels in the central nervous system (CNS) under baseline conditions in patients with chronic PTSD than in healthy subjects, and the higher levels correlated to symptom severity.[5]

Serotonin, a monoamine neurotransmitter that has various functions in the CNS including the regulation of mood, appetite, sleep, muscle contraction, and some cognitive functions including memory and learning, is also produced in the brainstem neurons that are located in the raphe nuclei. Serotonin neurons have many projections in the brain, however the ones most significant in PTSD are those associated to the neocortex, amygdala, and hippocampus. Different types of acute stress result in increased serotonin turnover in the medial prefrontal cortex, nucleus accumbens, amygdala and lateral hypothalamus in experimental animals.[6] However, exposure to repeated stress within a learned-helplessness model resulted in a decrease of serotonin release in the frontal cortex.[7] One possible theory is that this decrease in serotonin reflects serotonin depletion by continued release, however the same changes in norepinephrine are not documented with baseline CNS levels in PTSD subjects.[5] The importance of this "split" between norepinephrine and serotonin levels becomes important in later sections of this chapter.

One way in which Western physicians (particularly psychiatrists) treat PTSD is through pharmacological interventions with antidepressants that affect norepinephrine and serotonin. Selective Serotonin Reuptake Inhibitors (SSRIs), which block the reuptake of serotonin in the brain, and Serotonin and Norepinephrine Reuptake Inhibitors (SNRIs), which block serotonin and norepinephrine reuptake in the CNS, are the most frequently used pharmacological agents in the West for treating PTSD. Several double-blind placebo controlled clinical trials have shown mild to moderate responses for the elevating mood and anxiolytic (anxiety blocking) effects of these two classes of antidepressants.[8] Other medications that modulate/dampen sympathetic responses (central alpha and beta blockers), older classes of antidepressants (tricyclics), and atypical antipsychotic (that block certain types of serotonin receptors and some in this class have effects on the adrenal glands/HPA axis) have all been or are currently being studied for use in PTSD, but to date no single pharmacological agent has shown any type of superiority in ameliorating PTSD symptoms.[8] With respect to administering any type of substance deemed to possess medicinal value, appropriate clinical judgment is advised and should only be given within the context of the discipline in which a clinician/practitioner is licensed.

Psychology of PTSD

Sigmund Freud (1856–1939) was an Austrian neurologist who is considered to be the founder of modern psychiatry, as well as the

creator of classic psychoanalysis.[8] Freud is renowned for his theories of the unconscious mind and defining various psychological defense mechanisms utilized by humans to defend against stressful experiences, most notably repression.[9] He laid the foundation for the clinical practice of psychoanalysis (talk therapy), and is infamous for his redefinition of sexual desire as the primary motivational energy of human life.[8] Perhaps he is best known around the world for dream interpretation as a source of insight into unconscious desires, and among psychiatric academic circles his legacy of theories regarding transference in the therapeutic relationship (where a patient "transfers" his or her own previous perceptions of past relationships onto the therapist) and therapeutic techniques including the use of free association, endures to this day.[8] Although many of Freud's ideas are now considered flawed and antiquated (even Freud himself predicted that when knowledge of brain physiology increased many of his theories would be revised), his groundbreaking methods and theories still hold an important place in clinical psychoanalysis and psychodynamic approaches.

I am writing this section with an additional cautionary statement that practitioners unlicensed in psychotherapy should not attempt to perform "talk therapy" with their PTSD clients/patients unless they are trained and licensed to do so. Psychotherapy is a complex art that typically requires years of training under guided supervision. This section is being included to provide a better understanding of what commonalities are occurring between the biological and energy disturbances associated with PTSD, and to aide in the understanding of the interplay between the three. If it is evident that a patient's psychopathology is interfering with energy treatments that a practitioner is employing, then an appropriate referral to a qualified professional should be made. The term "psychotherapy" is as general a term as "martial art" because there are various different styles and approaches in achieving a desired therapeutic response. For example, "classic psychoanalysis" (where a patient comes into a therapist's office and "lays on a couch" to free associate) is but one style of psychotherapy that usually takes a substantial number of "sessions" in order for a patient to achieve insight into his or her psychological structure that is likely causing them clinically significant distress.

One of the best books I have read on psychotherapy is authored by

Nancy McWilliams (*Psychoanalytic Diagnosis: Understanding Personality Structure in the Clinical Process*, 1994) and I recommend it as required reading for any practitioner who desires a genuine understanding of human character structure. McWilliams does an eloquent job supporting her premise that humans are operating on two distinct and interactive dimensions: "a developmental level of personality organization, and a defensive style(s) within that level" [i.e. what is the person's pathology (psychotic, "neurotic", borderline, adaptive) and what is the person's character (antisocial, paranoid, depressive, anxious, schizoid)]?[9] Although she does not delve deeply into Acute Stress Reactions and PTSD, viewing patients with the above mindset significantly aides in identifying a patient's core psychological organization, as well as defensive styles he or she is using to cope with their illness.[9] Defensive styles typically observed in PTSD are being highlighted in these next few sections in order to give the practitioner of whatever discipline being utilized (whether it be herbal medicine, acupuncture, Reiki, qi-gong, meridian work, or Western psychiatry) a better psychological understanding of the patients he or she will be treating.

Freud originally classified defense mechanisms ("styles" in which human beings use their minds to deal with stress) into narcissistic, immature, neurotic and mature.[8] Others have simplified this classification as either primary (or primitive) and secondary (or higher-order) processes.[9] It is beyond the scope of this chapter to delve into defining the major and minor defenses that have been identified in various psychological schools of thought (somewhere near fifty). The most important ones that are relevant for combat veterans with PTSD are avoidance, numbing, repression, denial, acting out, dissociation (derealization and depersonalization), projection, and identifying with the aggressor.[10] Many psychological theories abound about what causes PTSD, from classical and operant conditioning (where the original traumatic event involves a learned association of the emotional trauma to the traumatic event and when triggers are encountered the trauma is relived, anxiety occurs, and avoidance/numbing can successfully defend against future anxiety, thus are reinforced)[10] to the behavioral model of combined associations that give meaning to the traumatic event (which stresses the importance of the "fear structure" that skew/shift core beliefs

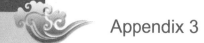
to "I am never safe", "I can be killed anytime", "the world is not fair", "I am all alone" and invariably leads to incomplete processing of the trauma and continued feelings of helplessness).[10,11]

Anger (particularly in combat veterans) plays an important role in PTSD psychodynamics, as survivors often hold intense rage towards those they deem responsible for their trauma and frequently project this strong emotion onto others who are connected to the traumatic event, thus intensifying their anxiety.[10] In my practice this is seen all too often with combat veterans who hold an entire institution as co-contributors to their traumatization (i.e. his of her country's "Army"). In order to diminish the power of intense fear and anger in their psyche, PTSD sufferers frequently identify with their aggressor to dispel helplessness and diminish the power their perceived victimization holds over their psyche, only to have intense survivor guilt (especially if deaths occurred during the traumatic event) about allying themselves with their aggressors.[10] They may use denial to empower their psyche that their psychological integrity remained intact despite suffering a trauma, or act out in outbursts of anger and rage to dispel their shattered worldview. Repression (a motivated forgetting or ignoring) is a basic higher-order defense and is commonly misconstrued as a primary defense mechanism for PTSD as a means of avoiding the intense fear and horror that a life threatening event would have on one's ego, however McWilliams argues that this psychological response to trauma is more consistent with dissociation (movement into an altered state of consciousness when one is distressed).[9]

Sometimes mistaken for the psychic defense of "splitting", dissociation differs because it is associated with amnesia; either with the behavior, emotions, physical sensations, or knowledge of the traumatic event[9] (please refer to the above definition of PTSD). However, the essence of dissociation is a "splitting" from ones own awareness of their reality. It is the primary defense used in "split" or "multiple personality disorder" (now called dissociative identity disorder) and was once considered rarely used as a primary defense.[9] However, to experienced clinicians it is being recognized as a primary coping style for traumatic exposures. There is evidence that the more a person is traumatized, the greater the probability they will employ this defense (i.e. single event traumas like rape or assault are more easily remembered than repetitive traumas like front-line combat or torture).[12] For over a hundred years, scores of combat veterans have reported delayed recall in traumatic events they have experienced. That fact that this occurred decades before the now common practice of compensating disabled veterans for psychological injury lends credibility that delayed recall is a valid phenomenon. The more one is traumatized the harder it becomes to integrate an experience without dissociation.[9] I have had thousands of soldiers tell me during a session, "I'm going crazy", "I'm remembering things that I didn't know I went through", "I feel intense rage and fear for no reason", "I can remember my buddy dying in my arms and I have no feeling for it, I've become a monster". These statements speak to highly dissociative states that support the biological model of a disconnect "splitting" between amygdala and hippocampal functioning, as affect states are recalled without provocation and have no "narrative memory" associated with it, and the narrative memory can be recalled with no "emotional memory".

Dissociate states have the potential to be extremely disabling, and many combat-related PTSD patients utilize self-medication with drugs and alcohol in an attempt to either reinforce avoidance and numbing, or evoke an emotional response (i.e. crying or releasing rage). I have sat through many lectures from various experts in the field of combat-related PTSD, and several have given convincing arguments that every patient diagnosed with PTSD possesses two character traits that, if not addressed in therapy, will allow PTSD to continue indefinitely. The first trait is avoidance; the second is an inability to let go of highly activating emotional states. These same lecturers have argued that a "shift in schema" (i.e. their world view) has occurred and this invariably involves a state of learned helplessness. Various treatment modalities have been suggested to assimilate the traumatic experience(s) into a patient's psyche in order to achieve remission (flooding, cognitive behavioral therapy, affect regulation, graded exposure, brief-supportive, insight-oriented, psychodynamic therapy, logotherapy) and are too numerous for the purposes of this chapter to explain in great detail. Many are beyond the scope of an acupuncturist, herbalist, Reiki, or qi-gong practitioner to utilize. However, providers of the above mentioned disciplines should have a basic understanding of PTSD psychology because re-traumatizing

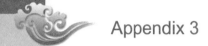

the patient should be avoided. Allow the patient to be the gatekeeper of what experiences they wish to share.

The Energy of PTSD

As a board certified psychiatrist in the United States, this is perhaps the most challenging section to write about because there is a common misconception that energy work in the Western practice of medicine is ineffectual, anecdotal, and lacking with respect to the gold standard of double blind, placebo controlled trials. However, if one takes the time to perform a thorough review of the literature on qi-gong, acupuncture, herbology, and Reiki, it becomes overwhelmingly clear that studies in this field are numerous and convincing. The Chinese have performed hundreds of studies regarding the therapeutic value of qi-gong (a practice working with "qi" or the "universal energy" that flows through a body, and is often confused with tai-chi); however most of them are published in Chinese, thus making it difficult for Western clinicians to access and appreciate their validity. I personally have not read any of these published qi-gong studies (mainly because I cannot read Chinese) but a qi-gong practitioner experienced in the treatment of thousands of Reflex Sympathetic Dystrophy patients [abbreviated RSD, and as of 1995 RSD was renamed to Complex Regional Pain Syndrome (CRPS)] educated me about their existence and has a series of translations that I look forward to reading. Unfortunately, as this book goes to press I have not yet been able to familiarized myself with the Chinese qi-gong clinical evidence/trials, so I must refer the reader to previous chapters in this book that have been authored by qi-gong experts.

My experience in energy work is mainly with the classes I took in Reiki, and the resources I've read by Caroline Myss, Ph.D. (a five-time *New York Times* best selling author and internationally renowned speaker in the fields of human consciousness, spirituality and mysticism, health, and energy medicine) and Bruce Lipton, PH. D., author of *The Biology of Belief*. Joe Chang, a licensed diplomate in acupuncture (Dipl. O.M., L.Ac) that holds a Masters of Acupuncture and Oriental Medicine (MAOM) and a main contributing author to this textbook who primarily treats PTSD patients at the major military instillation where we both work also provided me first-hand testimonials about his experience using acupuncture to treat PTSD. I will refer the reader to the chapters authored by Joe and other acupuncturists for a better conceptualization of the energy meridians that are being utilized for the treatment of PTSD.

Joe's findings correlate beautifully to the Eastern-based chakra system Caroline Myss, PH.D., uses as the foundation to conceptualize energy imbalances as it relates to medical disease presentations.[13] In her book, *Anatomy of the Spirit,* she brilliantly interweaves the seven christian sacraments, seven sacred kabala spiritual truths, and the hindu chakra system (which contains seven "energy" centers) and uses them to outline a roadmap of human spiritual development. As I keep reiterating, it is beyond the scope of this textbook chapter to elaborate on all the nuances of physical and psychological disease as it relates to energy imbalances, especially using Caroline Myss's model, however the energy centers pertinent to PTSD will be covered briefly in order to give the reader a better understanding of meridian and chakra imbalances that typically occur with PTSD. Dr. Myss states that "the chakra system is an archetypal depiction of individual maturation through seven distinct phases" and opines that the basis for all psychological illnesses stems from disorders of the first (or root) chakra.[13] The "chakras" are conceptualized as vertically aligned energy centers that start from the base of the spine and ascend to the crown of the head, and as each energy center is mastered (per Myss's theory each one contains a universal spiritual life-lesson) knowledge of personal and spiritual power increases.[13] Starting from the root and finishing with the crown, these life-lessons are: all is one, honor one another, honor one-self, love is divine power, surrender personal will to divine will, seek only the truth, and live in the present moment.[13] In addition to the life-lesson contained within each chakra she subcategorized each one to a location, energy connection to the physical body, energy connection to the emotional/mental body, symbolic/ perceptual connection, primary fears, primary strengths, and the kabala/ sacrament connection.[13]

As a master-level Reiki practitioner, I was taught the basic structures of the seven chakras, what organs they govern, and the physical manifestations in the body associated with disharmony in each one. Caroline Myss's above conceptualization has likely influenced some of the

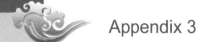

mainstream Reiki practitioner's understanding of this concept, and I will do my best to credit her teachings where appropriate. The major chakras I will expand upon are chakras one, two, three, and four, with minor references to five, six, and seven.

Myss stated that the root (first) chakra is the foundation of emotional and mental health. She calls it the tribal chakra as it represents a group identity (either family unit or organization).[13] The emotional issues include (but are not limited to) safety in numbers and social law and order. Physical dysfunctions can include chronic low back pain and depression.[13] When a combat related trauma is suffered, the patient likely belongs to the tribal culture of a military organization, and my experience with treating this group reveals that repeated combat exposures shatters his or hers faith in this institution. One of the major structures the second chakra governs is the sexual organs, and in my experience this chakra's energy is the first and most easily identifiable in a normally developing child. Perhaps this is why Freud originally thought all drives were based in sexual desires. Some of the major emotional and mental issues Myss associates with this chakra are blame, guilt, power, and control. Thousands of PTSD patients I have treated espouse endless blame and guilt for the traumas they have suffered, and in my opinion, feelings of extreme helplessness (i.e. loss of power) start at this level as well. A vast majority of PTSD patients report low back pain and sciatica issues, which could be related to the energy dysfunction at these two levels, in addition to the normal "wear and tear" of a foot soldier.

The third chakra (Myss states this one as the "personal power chakra")[13] is associated with many corresponding physical structures, but the most relevant ones include the liver, kidney, adrenal glands, and spleen. Joe has stated that he most frequently sees an excess pattern in the liver channel, and this corresponds with Myss's mental and emotional association to fear. Traumatic events cause autonomic arousal and would explain the excess pattern in this channel, and also correspond biologically to the high CNS norepinephrine levels found in baseline samples of PTSD patients.[4] He also noted that after he balances the liver and heart channels he frequently identifies a deficiency pattern in the kidney and spleen channels. Such a finding suggests decreased trust, decreased personal honor, and decreased self-esteem/respect/confidence that PTSD patients report, and correlate to the other emotional and mental issues that Myss diagram as being governed by this chakra.[13] This simultaneous excess and deficiency state speaks to a "split" within the liver channel, and within the third chakra.

The biological correlation to the fourth chakra corresponds with the physical location of the heart, and Myss states that mental and emotional issues at this level deal with love and hate, grief and anger, resentment and bitterness, forgiveness and compassion, and hope and trust. Intense fear and rage that accompanies PTSD correlates to the excess patterns Joe has reported in the heart channel, and in conjunction with the deficiency states documented in the liver channel, it becomes even more evident that there is a "split" in the energy flow between the second, third, and fourth chakras. The decreased energy and fatigue he noted could also be due to adrenal dysfunction, and this energy finding biologically correlates to the clinical studies done on HPA axis dysregulation mentioned above. In addition to intense fear, grief for fallen comrades can be simultaneously occurring, as well as resentment and bitterness towards the perpetrators of their trauma, making trust and forgiveness more difficult to achieve.

It is worth mentioning the fifth chakra because addiction is associated with this energy center, indicating issues with choice, strength of will, faith and knowledge, and the capacity to make decisions. Myss has identified these as the emotional and mental issues of the fifth chakra.[13] The sixth chakra governs the physical structures of the brain and nervous system, and Myss states that, among other mental and emotional issues, truth and the ability to learn from one's experiences are inherent life-lessons within this level. The "split" between second and third chakra energies, in addition to the "split" within the third chakra itself, with combined excess patterns of the third and fourth energy centers, "confuses" the brain and makes learning from experience difficult. Also, repeated trauma makes dissociation more common as a psychiatric defense (see above) thus further deepening the split that occurs within the sixth chakra itself (i.e. the disconnect between amygdala and hippocampal functioning),[12] and between chakras two through four. Chakras two through four are also in an imbalanced state with the sixth one. This "split" disrupts the process of assimilating traumatic experiences and assigning meaning to them, which is a treatment goal for most psychotherapy patients.

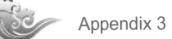

Joe has stated that when he balances the heart channel, soldiers frequently report decreased nightmares. Like muscle memory, "heart memory" circulating within the fourth chakra could finally be making a connection to the sixth (brain) chakra, thus allowing for integration of traumatic experiences within the human energy system and enhance the psychological stage of learning from one's trauma and assigning meaning to it.

The seventh chakra corresponds physically to the skin and muscular/skeletal systems, and the emotional/mental issues that are required to achieve mastery at this level are the ability to trust life and see the larger pattern, as well as faith and inspiration. Of note, Caroline Myss worked with a Harvard trained neurosurgeon (C. Norman Shealy, M.D., Ph.D) and provided astonishingly accurate energy readings for his patients and the past/present experiences ongoing in their lives that were contributing to their illness. Harvard Medical School also funded two studies[14,15] (Hui et al. 2000, 2005) investigating the brain's response via functional magnetic resonance imaging (fMRI) when two commonly used acupuncture points were stimulated (LI4 on the hand and ST36 on the leg respectively). Startling results of decreased fMRI signals in several CNS structures, most notably the nucleus accumbens, amygdala, hippocampus, and ventral tegmental area, provided evidence that stimulation of traditional channel points also modulates the limbic system.[14,15] The exact nature as to what this modulation could be is explained above.

Integrating the Biology, Psychology, and Energy of PTSD

After evaluating and treating several thousand patients with PTSD, it becomes increasing clear that there is a disconnect within a patient's biological, psychological, and energetic makeup. Qualifying and quantifying this "split" is more readily achieved in the West using measurable outcomes (like the quantification of CNS neural transmitters in PTSD patients mentioned above[5,7]) than psychological or energy assessment and treatment modalities, however biological measures alone cannot account for all the symptoms experienced with PTSD. Conventional Western medicine is not the be-all and end-all for preventing, managing, and helping combat veterans extinguish their symptoms. I find myself making more referrals for alternative measures of treatment as the wars in Iraq and Afghanistan continue because medications and conventional psychotherapy (alone or together) do not produce results fast enough to return patients (who are soldiers) back to the work force. However, the DOD is finally giving energy medicine like Reiki, acupuncture, qi-gong, and massage a legitimate chance to succeed where pharmacological and psychological measures have failed. I was amazed when I discovered the Army base at which I practiced psychiatry started a program that incorporated Reiki, acupuncture, and massage into the treatment milieu for combat-related PTSD, and, that it was the second major base to do so (please refer to the forward I wrote for this book). A biological, psychological and energy based model for PTSD that incorporates Eastern and Western views is long overdue.

There is no cookie-cutter approach to any medical, psychological, or energy based disease. A foundational premise inherent to Western psychiatry residency programs is that no two patients are the same; each requires a tailored approach that will hopefully achieved a desired outcome with the resources available. For many in the West that means reaching for the prescription pad and writing for a medication, or scheduling a certain number of psychotherapy sessions to process and assimilate the trauma into the psyche, both with the same goal of increasing a patient's ability to cope and function. This is no different than the treatment goal of Eastern practices like herbology, qi-gong, Reiki, or acupuncture. In my opinion, the key to successful treatment of PTSD lies somewhere between the two, using a succinct and clear model of what the essence of the illness it, how it forms, what is the best method that will do the least harm to the patient, and how to sustain remission once positive results are achieved. One must keep in mind however, that no matter what level of expertise the clinician/practitioner is trying to effect change (either biological, psychological or energetically), PTSD has a recurring theme of a "split" within a patient's human architecture. To use a simple analogy, humans can be conceptualized as a three dimensional pyramid such that the base and the volume within it contains every single one of our experiences, from our first breath to the present moment, and each triangular face represents one aspect of the human trinity (body, mind or spirit).

I have come to believe the same truth that my experienced colleagues

shared with me when I was in residency; most, if not all of the patients I have evaluated with PTSD use dissociation and avoidance as their primary coping styles, and they have trouble letting go of their shattered world view (shift in "schema") that occurred as the result of their trauma. This invariably causes a "crack" or a "split" in the human pyramid, typically between the mind-spirit interface. Essentially this means that a person's particular belief or faith is "shattered" and is no longer congruent with their thinking. To help educate patients about this dichotomy within their human structure I simply pose the following question to them: "Is what you think to be true and what you know to be true now different since this unfortunate experience happened to you?" It is almost as if a light switch has been turned on inside their minds once they start to realize the divergence of their thinking and their beliefs. As humans, we all have fleeting thoughts that go through our minds on a daily basis and they are reflective of the internal dialogue a person has with one's own mind. A belief is a psychological state in which an individual hold a proposition or a premise to be true. In my opinion, belief borders on faith, which is an internal knowing that is a function of the soul. Like the "heart memory" of the fourth chakra I explained above, this knowing is not limited to one particular structure of the body (i.e. it is not confined to the brain, it flows through energy channels between the seven energy centers). Perhaps the chakras function as a center (like an organ) for divine truths (as Caroline Myss postulates) and the energy channels that acupuncturists, qi-gong and Reiki practitioners stimulate are like repairing energy channels connected to them (like a vascular surgeon repairing damaged blood vessels that are supplying a diseased organ).

Her experience as a medical intuitive led Caroline Myss to state one of the truest axioms I have read with respect to the validity of my profession and the importance that psychiatry holds in Eastern and Western medicine: our biography becomes our biology,[13] In reviewing the above biology section of PTSD, the take home message is that of a learned response (i.e. helplessness) having a biological consequence in the brain (serotonin levels that were initially elevated in high anxiety states decreased after learned helplessness)[7] yet norepinephrine level stayed the same. The implications are quite profound if thoroughly analyzed... *a change in thinking patterns caused a biological response in the brain.* If a change in thought patterns (one from empowerment to helplessness) can affect biochemical functioning of the brain, what other organ systems could be affected by our thinking? This very premise could account for the disruption in amygdala and hippocampal functioning as it relates to memory processing in the prefrontal cortex, and the disruption triggered by the psychological defense of dissociation (which commonly occurs with repeated trauma). This concept of thinking affecting our physical health and creating our physical reality is nothing new or revolutionary in some circles of Western thought. Dr. Bruce Lipton, a former medical school professor and research scientist in cell biology wrote about his experimental findings that genes and DNA do not control our biology; DNA is in fact controlled by signals from outside the cell, *including what we think and believe.*[16] What is revolutionary in this chapter is learning how to apply this knowledge to the PTSD patient population and recognizing that simultaneous use of Western and Eastern medicinal practices serves a valuable role in repairing the biological and psychological damage caused by destructive thought and belief patterns, and that using both can *dramatically increase* the rate of repair and recovery. This recovery might have eventually occurred merely by a patient changing one's thinking and beliefs, however the potential to accelerate the process using energy medicine holds true.

As I mentioned in the forward of this book, I came to Joe as a patient seeking relief from sympathetic mediated pain (also known as RSD/CRPS). I was already well aware of the association between one's thinking patterns and the biological effects they had on one's body. What I was able to appreciate and learn from Joe's acupuncture treatments is that my quality of life and pain improved considerably with Eastern treatments (in addition to performing acupuncture on me, Joe introduced me to Bob Deschner, a qi-gong practitioner who has worked with thousands of RSD patients). Although I am far from being cured, I have a new understanding of the nuances that exist in the three dimensional pyramid that embodies the human body-mind-spirit connection. Perhaps it was by design that PTSD is set apart from every other psychological disorder because one must experience a trauma in order to meet criteria for it, just like RSD/CRPS is set apart from all other medical diseases because one must experience a psychical injury/trauma in order to meet criteria for

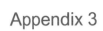

it. The essence of both diseases is autonomic dysfunction; PTSD from a psychological trauma and RDS from a physical trauma. But because of the mechanism of the trauma sustained involved different aspects of the human triad, one psychological and the other physical, a completely different disease presentation resulted (and I will expand upon this concept in the next section).

It is beyond the scope of this chapter to review RSD in its entirety; all that is required for the purposes of this book is that the manifestations of autonomic dysfunction from a physical injury (vascular changes, trophic changes, severe continuous pain, swelling, etc.) can have dramatic psychological effects with subtle physical findings. After several treatments with Joe and Bob I began to notice that my fatigue and mood improved, I could walk better, and the medications I took when I had a flare worked better. Joe stated he had similar reports from the thousands of soldiers he has treated (especially the perception about having to take less medication and when they were taken their efficacy improved). I was already seeing a Reiki practitioner and even received training from her on a master level. My results with Reiki were better than I received with conventional Western treatments, but it was the combination of adding acupuncture and qi-gong to reiki that produced the best results I've had to date. RSD is as psychically disabling as PTSD is psychological disabling. Any repeat trauma of the slightest nature (for RSD this could be a light touch or trivial fall; for PTSD this could be reminders in the form of loud noises or crowded places) can trigger massive flares of both, however employing Eastern traditions with conservative Western treatments shows potential for dramatically improving the rate of healing.

In a closing note, it is a commonly held psychiatric and global "tribal belief" (which is first chakra energy) that healing, especially from repeated traumatic exposures like those endured in front-line combat, takes a long time to achieve.[13] Believing it by many individuals and societies has considerably shaped the course of Western medicine and psychiatric practices, in the same manner that one's own belief and perception has a biological effects on one's own body. Psychiatrists as a whole tend to believe that the psychopathology which develops from severely traumatizing experiences takes years of psychotherapy and/or medications to heal. But as noted above, healing can occur quite rapidly if one believes it, and even more rapidly by combining biological, psychological and energy healing modalities. Myss states that, "By choosing to believe something, we breathe our breath into that belief, giving that belief authority [and] the length of the healing process becomes calibrated to the time that the tribal mind attunes to them."[13] She also goes on to state that, "If your spirit is strong enough to withdraw from the authority of a group belief, it is potentially strong enough to change your life..."[13]

I have come to regard spiritual and psychological fitness in the same manner physical fitness is attained. One must work at it with an established routine in order to achieve results. I have seen body builders increase inches of muscle mass in a relatively short amount of time (within two weeks) and without the use of steroids, just based on the method in which they performed their workouts. Psychological and energy fitness should be no different, and by rapidly affirming healthier thought patterns and employing traditions of qi-gong, Reiki, and acupuncture (that help open up energy channels in the body) the connections between the body, mind and spirit can be strengthened, reestablished, and reinforced, and health may be rapidly achieved.

Cautionary Statement

Other chapters of this book cover the topic of compassion fatigue, and as a psychiatrist I tend to view such an occurrence with the Freudian perspective of "transference". Care providers for a patient population with severe symptoms (like PTSD patients at a military installation) are increasingly reporting a syndrome known as "compassion fatigue". Many are providers with no prior combat exposures or traumatic experiences, yet are reporting experiences similar to their patients' (combat-related flashbacks, nightmares, intrusive thoughts, increased startle response, irritability, sleep disturbance, and avoidant behaviors). Classical psychoanalytic thought would argue that transference and/or projective identification is occurring (where a patient is projecting his or her experiences onto the caretaker and the caretaker is internalizing these projections on an unconscious or conscious level). There are always risks associated with every type of treatment modality, even with just "talking" to a patient (as occurs in psychotherapy), although it would seem that the

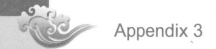

risk in this circumstance goes both ways. Every effort should be made by those treating high acuity, high volume, and/or severely symptomatic patient populations to remain centered in their discipline, find healthy and creative physical outlets, build a strong social support network, and take appropriate breaks/vacations as needed.

I risk certain criticism for sharing some of my own experiences in this realm because psychiatrists are grounded in the belief that this type of knowledge should be kept from patients (i.e. the less a patient knows about his or her physician, the less it interferes with the healing process). I refer critics to the above quote from Caroline Myss. I share this experience with the reader because I can find no better example or case history that will help illustrate or deepen one's understanding of my proposed model for the three dimensional body-mind-spirit pyramid that forms the basis for human existence and how PTSD effects it. While serving a seven month tour in Iraq I sustained an injury to my right ankle when dismounting from a Black Hawk. The injury never healed and the pain remained localized to my ankle, but quickly spread to my calf. After returning to the States the pain spread to my thigh and groin, and eventually to right trunk, arm and face. This is a classic presentation for RSD. The sympathetic nervous system, by unknown mechanisms, "takes control" over pain perception, and is pathological. The slightest injury or stimulation can result in excruciating pain. This is how I came to meet Joe, because RSD/CRPS by nature is difficult to treat and conventional Western medicine knows little on how to effectively manage it. However, before I was injured I was well aware of the connection between thinking patterns and how they affect one's biology. I was steadfast in my belief structure that if only I intended and thought of health, I would have it.

But what I failed to recognize was the effect that seeing thousands of severely distressed PTSD patients would have on me on an unconscious level, and how it contributed to this non-healing injury of mine. It wasn't until I was watching an episode of one of my favorite television series that I realize the effects my medical practice was having on my thought patterns. The episode involved a dream sequence in which the main character was enacting a desert combat scenario, although he had never been in combat. The vehicle he was a passenger in was hit by an explosive device. This was a scenario I have heard and visualized thousands of times from the soldiers I cared for, only I didn't realize that this experience had entrenched itself in my psyche. Watching this dream sequence on TV made me burst into tears. I began to relive in my mind many of the stories I had heard from soldiers I had treated and, at that moment, I was experiencing them as if they were my own. My underlying faith and beliefs about the body-mind-spirit connection were strong, but my thinking had changed, thus causing a "split" in the spirit-mind interface (as opposed to PTSD, which is a "split" or "crack" in the pyramid's structure at the mind-spirit interface). Both PTSD and RSD have autonomic dysfunction as a core feature. But because of the mechanisms involved-in my case a strong belief structure with shifted thought patterns-a more physiological effect manifested in my body. The message I took away from this realization is that our beliefs are more powerful than the way we think, even on a physical level. I was having mild success with my injury by changing my thought patterns and decreasing my volume of patients, but doing energy work with Reiki, qi-gong, and acupuncture is increased my energy fitness, as well as furthering my understanding of PTSD and the power of transference. By opening up energy channels and balancing energy centers, the speed with which dysfunctional thought patterns are changed to healthier ones can be accelerated in order to achieve physical and psychological health at a faster rate.

Conclusion

PTSD is a psychological disorder that has provided a unique opportunity to view the overlay between biological, psychological, and energy processes that are occurring in humans. It aided in the development of a pyramidal concept for the body-mind-spirit model that fully encompasses human architectural design. Western medicine is finally starting to embrace Eastern medicine as a valid treatment for this disabling psychological illness, in large part because the DOD has started pilot programs at two major military installations. The results appear promising and cost effective. The world stage is being set to combine Eastern and Western treatment modalities on a global scale, which can only serve to strengthen and deepen our understanding of human physiology and the role psychology and spiritual fitness plays in sustaining physical health. A combined approach is a wise approach so

long as the patient is fully educated and informed about the risks, benefits, alternatives, and potential side effects about the treatment modality being utilized to treat their condition. Patients who are staunch in their resistance to undergo Eastern or Western treatment options should not be forced to do so as this may further deepen dysfunctional belief and thought patterns about their condition. However, most patients whom I've encountered (myself included) have benefited immensely from embracing Eastern styles of thought and medicinal practices. At this point in time, the potential benefit in applying a combined Eastern and Western treatment approach to other psychiatric and medical diseases outweighs the risk, and every attempt should be made to further study this avenue of healing.

Appendix 4
Reiki Healing for Soldiers with PTSD

Reiki healing methods are often very beneficial in the treatment of soldiers suffering with PTSD. The benefits that we describe here are presented according to an anecdotal model as opposed to any kind of scientific analysis. However, based on these experiential results, interest in clinical research on the effects of Reiki as applied to PTSD is growing substantially.

The term Post-Traumatic Stress Disorder (PTSD) was first used as a psychiatric diagnosis in 1980. Although the term was initially applied to survivors of sexual assault and other violent crimes, it later became strongly associated with the emotional and behavioral symptom patterns seen in many combat veterans from the Vietnam War. However, this certainly was not the first time that military personnel experienced the severe negative after-effects of being wounded, nearly dying, killing others, or witnessing all the horrors of war. This same reactive and difficult to treat condition was called "the soldier's heart" during the Civil War, "shell shock" in WWI, and then "battle fatigue" in WWⅡ. PTSD symptom patterns have been reported in warriors of many cultures and eras.

PTSD has many different definitions depending on one's point of view, as well as a very specific set of formal criteria in the DSM-IV. It is often defined as a type of anxiety disorder, a mental illness caused by an enduring reaction to exposure to a terrifying event or events, with specific consequences—hyper-arousal, avoidance of stimuli related to the events and intrusive memories or reliving of all or parts of the memories. This is a very narrow definition. Using a whole person model, PTSD is much more than a mental issue because it affects every aspect of the person: body, mind, emotions, and spirit.

Physically, soldiers with PTSD usually report severe pain in parts of their body or throughout their entire body. Most also have sleep disorders

and often nightmares. While some physical reactions are side effects of combat wounds, others are clearly the consequences of constant neural and biochemical stress responses impacting on the nervous system and the body. For example, gastrointestinal symptoms resembling irritable bowel disorder are quite common in soldiers returning from Iraq and Afghanistan. Elevated resting heart rates and blood pressures in young, physically fit soldiers are a diagnostic problem for military health care providers. Headaches can be chronic, even without the all too common post-concussion symptoms seen in soldiers who have been exposed to blasts. Unexplained sleep apnea symptoms are also common. Sexual dysfunction, usually from loss of desire, is reported frequently.

Mentally, these soldiers who have witnessed the horrors of war can experience severe anxiety, depression, and a sense of being helpless and hopeless. Existential conflicts over loss of meaning, with a kind of uncaring cynicism, are often reported. Many believe that only other soldiers can understand them, and pessimism about the future is common. Memories of traumatic events are often fragmented, and symptoms of dissociation often appear. Concentration and attention may also be impaired.

Emotionally, combat personnel with PTSD can be out of balance at opposite ends of the feeling spectrum. Some lock down their emotional heart so they are unable to feel normal human emotions; this often results in feeling disconnected from others, including family members and loved ones. Many swing to the opposite end of the emotional continuum and are given to easily triggered violent outbursts of anger and rage. Both of these emotional conditions cause great difficulty in family relationships, friendships and employment. Depressive symptoms are almost universal, as is a generalized anxiety about safety.

At the spiritual level, many soldiers report losing their faith and being disillusioned about their prior religious beliefs. Other soldiers with severe PTSD have received a trauma so intense that the experience is as if an important aspect of themselves is actually leaving their bodies. In metaphysical terms, this is called "soul loss" or a wounding of the soul. This affliction has been described in many ancient cultures where shamanic practitioners are called upon to restore lost parts of the self or soul. Modern medicine has no equivalent practices, but soldiers and other traumatized persons continue to report this phenomenon.

Those with soul loss can have a vacant look to their eyes, which is often described as the "thousand yard stare." Some accurately describe this condition of soul loss by saying, "The lights are on but there's nobody home." Edward Tick, Ph.D. writes in *War and the Soul*, "In the presence of overwhelming life-threatening violence, the soul—the true self—flees. What is called 'soul loss' is an extreme psycho-spiritual condition beyond what psychologists commonly call dissociation. With body and soul separated, a person is trapped in a limbo where past and present intermingle with little differentiation or continuity. Nothing feels right until body and soul rejoin."

Because PTSD affects soldiers physically, mentally, emotionally, and spiritually, it only seems logical that PTSD treatment must also address these same four levels. Many complementary and alternative methods are known to treat all four levels of being; these include acupuncture, yoga, qigong, body therapies such as massage and cranial sacral work, and bio-energy therapies, of which Reiki healing is a very common example.

What is Reiki Healing?

William Rand, a Reiki Master Teacher who has a center in Michigan and teaches all over the world, has a comprehensive explanation of Reiki on his website www.reiki.org. There he states the following: "Reiki is now practiced throughout North and South America, Europe, New Zealand, Australia, Japan, India and other parts of the world. There are now an estimated 1,000,000 Reiki Masters with as many as 4,000,000 people having been initiated into Reiki throughout the world. A study done in 2007 by the National Health Interview Survey indicates that 1.2 million adults and 161,000 children received one or more sessions of energy healing therapy such as Reiki in the previous year. According to the American Hospital Association, in 2007, 15% or over 800 American hospitals offered Reiki as part of hospital services."

There is a growing body of research available on Reiki. The Center for Reiki Research has created a website to promote the scientific awareness of Reiki by providing a current list of evidence based research published in peer reviewed journals along with summaries of each. The website also has a list of hospitals, medical clinics, and hospice programs where Reiki sessions are offered. Thousands of licensed health care practitioners such as nurses, doctors, physical therapists, massage therapists, psychologists,

and social workers have completed advanced Reiki training and integrate this healing modality into their work with patients. In the research studies, overall summaries of findings report that Reiki significantly reduces stress, decreases the amount of pain medication required, improves sleep and appetite, and accelerates the healing process of injuries and wounds. Reiki is often used along side traditional cancer treatments and this Japanese healing modality has also been reported to reduce many of the unwanted side effects of radiation and drugs, including chemotherapy.

C. Norman Shealy, M.D. Ph.D., founder of the American Holistic Medical Association had this to say about Reiki: "Reiki is one of the leading and safest energy medicine approaches. The study summaries provided by the Center for Reiki Research are the best source for information on Reiki research."

The Japanese healing modality called "Reiki" is one of many types of what the US NIH National Institute of Complementary and Alternative Medicine (NICAM) calls "biofield therapies." It involves the use of focused mental intention and the energy field of the practitioner in order to bring the Universal Energy called "Reiki" to bear on the person being healed.

Reiki has a long and complex history, first in Japan and later throughout the world. Traditional Reiki practices remain active in Japan and a separate, derived form is practiced in the West. American practitioners usually trace their lineage to Hawayo Takata, a Japanese woman in Hawaii, who brought the technique from Japan just before WW II. She trained a number of Master practitioners (usually listed as 22 individuals) who then spread the technique throughout the United States and Europe.

Reiki training is a multi-level process with practitioner students initiated through three levels, including a Master level for those that will teach the method and pass it on to their students. Reiki is seen as an initiation process rather than training because the Master actually influences the energy field of the student to allow them to tap into the universal Reiki energy by choice. Additional training involves learning how to apply Reiki energy treatments to others and oneself, a code of ethics, and how to use visualizations and images to further direct this energy.

A Reiki session commonly involves the subject lying on a massage table while the practitioner moves their hands on, over or around the person's body. There are standard hand positions for the basic treatment, with varied hand positions for advanced treatments. The practitioner may or may not touch the subject. Recipients often report heat emanating from the practitioner's hands or, in some cases, a cooling. Some have positive results objectively and do not experience anything subjectively. Most subjects experience profound relaxation and a sense of peace and inner quiet during the session. Pain relief is quite common. Physical effects accumulate over a series of sessions, seeming to reflect a speeding up or deepening of normal healing responses. Occasional profound and immediate emotional and physical effects reflect the potential for a dramatic wholistic impact of Reiki treatments.

Reiki theory includes the core concept that the Reiki energy is holistic and thus impacts all levels of the person—addressing mental, emotional, physical and spiritual domains. As such, it may be used to address any form of human dysfunction. Some authorities call Reiki the perfect "general purpose" healthcare modality, offering help for virtually any distress, disorder or symptom. It can be considered as "spiritual" in a generic sense, but Reiki involves no doctrines, creeds, or religious practices.

Case Studies

Lu Whitaker was first initiated into Reiki about twenty years ago. She is now a Reiki Master as well as a Master Teacher and has trained hundreds of other Reiki practitioners. For the last 18 months, she has been a part of a unique clinic at a US Army Hospital that provides integrative medicine treatment of combat-related PTSD in active duty soldiers. In addition to the usual psychological and mind/body treatments, the clinic uses massage, acupuncture, yoga and tai-chi, as well as Reiki in a synergistic healing program. During a series of interviews for this article Lu explained the Reiki process she uses with the soldiers.

The Reiki sessions are done individually in a private room with soothing music playing softly in the background. After removing their shoes, the soldiers lie fully clothed on my massage table. I review their charts to see where they have the most physical pain. I also ask them where they want me to focus. I place my

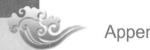

hands wherever the men or women have physical pain. Sometimes I touch the body and other times I hold my hands a few inches away. I do very little talking since the goal of the session is to let the spiritual energy do the healing. All of the soldiers can feel a gentle heat that comes from my hands into their body. I always tell them, "This is not my energy you are feeling. The energy you are receiving comes from the highest source—whatever you call that in your belief system: a Higher Power, Spirit, God, the Universe." The Reiki energy seems to have a beneficial effect regardless of their belief system.

At this time, each soldier in our program receives one Reiki session each week for three weeks. Before their first session they are simply instructed to attend and "be open" because this treatment that has had many good results for soldiers with PTSD. Rarely do the soldiers know what to expect since the majority have never heard of Reiki. Mostly they are quite curious before their first session begins. Afterwards many report, "That's not at all what I expected." I can safely say that no one has ever gotten off my table and said, "I don't feel any better."

This work with the soldiers is very rewarding. "There's a fulfillment that happens with each session that is more than what I've experienced with other populations. I have such gratitude for getting to do this work. It is such a blessing in my life."

Case 1

Restored Sleep

John is one of the soldiers who returned from his second tour in Iraq with severe body pain that was eventually diagnosed as fibromyalgia. After being in intense combat for months, he also became hypervigilant and developed a sleep disorder attributed to his state of hyperarousal. He had not been able to sleep in years, existing on what he called "catnaps". Lu described the results of his first Reiki session:

John entered a deep state of relaxation within minutes of starting the Reiki session. He fell into a sound sleep and slept the entire session. At the end of our time together I had to gently nudge his shoulder to wake him up. He woke without any startle response. As he sat up he spontaneously announced, "I feel more rested than I have since the bombing of the towers on 9/11 (eight years earlier). And my fibro pain in my feet is 50% improved." When he returned the next week he reported that after his first

Reiki session he slept through the night for the first time in seven years. He was a very happy soldier.

Case 2

Improved Pain after Surgery

Soldiers with physical pain consistently report to Lu that their pain level becomes reduced by nearly 50% during a Reiki treatment. One soldier came to see Lu a few weeks after receiving jaw surgery.

Here he describes the results of her first Reiki session:

This young soldier told me his jaw pain was a 10 on a scale of 1 to 10. He had been in constant pain for two weeks. He did not want me to touch his jaw, so I held my hands on each side of his head, not touching his face; I kept my hands about an inch away. Within several minutes he reported that he could feel heat coming from my hands. We did almost no talking so he could relax and maintain his focus on the healing energy (the heat) coming into both sides of his face. As we finished the session he sat up with a shocked look on his face. He announced, "I can't believe this. My pain went from a 10 to a 4. This is the best I've felt since my surgery."

Case 3

Improved Headache Pain

After returning from the war, the majority of soldiers with PTSD report ongoing headaches from mild to severe. Reiki is very effective in reducing their headache pain.

Lu described working with a woman soldier who had experienced numerous explosions in Iraq.

A young woman soldier with PTSD told me she had a "splitting headache" as she settled herself on my table. She described her pain level as a 12 on a scale from 1 to 10. She added that she had been suffering with headache pain for several years and that her numerously prescribed pain medications brought little relief. I kept my hands several inches from her head the whole session, and I could feel a lot of heat flowing through my hands. She quickly relaxed and went to sleep as I continued to move my hands in different positions around her head.

When I woke her at the end of the session she said with great surprise, "My pain is completely gone. I can hardly believe it! Nobody could have

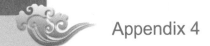

convinced me this could even happen." Then I told her, "Well, you're not the first one. Most of the soldiers I work on have headaches. After our Reiki session their headaches are either completely gone or greatly relieved".

Case 4

A Deep Sense of Peace

Many of the soldiers with PTSD are experiencing a spiritual crisis–although they might not identify it as such. Many are angry with God. They ask questions like: "If there is a God, why am I seeing my friends die in front of me? Why was I saved when my buddies died? If there is a God why does He let a war happen?" Some are atheists who don't even believe in God. Lu explained how often Reiki works with soldiers in a spiritual crisis.

Almost every soldier who lies on my table relaxes physically, becomes very quiet, and feels a deep sense of peace as he or she receives the Reiki energy. Many use the words "comforting" or "nurturing" to describe the energy. One woman announced, "I just want to stay here and feel the comfort and the safety of this experience. I don't want it to end." Another young male soldier said at the end of his first session, "I feel safe—like I haven't felt in years." All the soldiers seem to experience this deep sense of peace regardless of their belief system. The anger seems to dissipate for those who are angry with God. This sense of deep peace is a step towards alleviating the hyperarousal seen in most soldiers with PTSD.

Case 5

Spiritual Awakening

After receiving even a few Reiki treatments, significant minorities of soldiers with PTSD experience a type of spiritual awakening. In these cases, the Reiki energy seems to forge a connection between body and soul; light comes back into the eyes of a soldier who previously displayed "the thousand yard stare." Hopelessness about ever healing from PTSD is replaced by hope when the soul wounding becomes healed. When this happens, it is a gift of grace since the soldier has no knowledge about how to heal himself at this level. Lu described the transformation of a soldier who experienced "soul retrieval" after only three Reiki sessions.

When David first got onto my table, he was filled with an anger that he thought was entirely justified. He was angry with his wife who had recently filed for divorce. He was angry about his back pain and his injured knees. He was angry at the whole world and often flew into rages with no warning. His children were afraid of him because they never knew when he might explode.

Something shifted within David after his first Reiki session, and his anger simply evaporated. Miraculously, within weeks he made peace with all the problems in his life, including accepting his divorce as a good thing. He also became highly sensitive to the emotions of others—including his two children ages sixteen and three. After his three Reiki sessions he seemed better able to understand both children and better communicate with them. He decided to become the custodial parent and is now enjoying a healthy relationship with them.

David's back and knee pain diminished significantly. He also began to experience psychic phenomenon such as precognitive visions and dreams, spiritual visions, and mental telepathy. He spontaneously developed the ability to seen the energy fields (auras) around people and read their energies.

This young soldier felt motivated to seek further Reiki experiences. He enrolled in Reiki training and began using the Reiki energy for self-healing. He completely alleviated his sleep problems by doing Reiki on himself every night as he went to bed. David also uses Reiki on his two children who love receiving this healing energy from their Dad. He reports that both children are calm and peaceful even though the family is in the throes of a divorce. David himself seems to have a very peaceful heart—it is now filled with "the peace that passes all understanding."

Conclusion

In this brief summary, the application of Reiki healing to soldiers and others with PTSD is only partially described. In many settings across the USA and the world (hospitals, Veteran's clinics, pain centers, and psychiatric treatment settings), Reiki practitioners are applying these ancient tools, and their patients are reporting relief. Scientists continue to seek understanding of the mechanisms involved. As noted above, Reiki is a technique that restores health and balance at all levels impacted by trauma—physical, mental, emotional, and spiritual. The continued growth of the use of energy healing with PTSD patients can only be expected to continue.

Key References

1. Kessler RC, Sonnega A, Bromet E, et al. Posttraumatic stress disorder in the National Comorbidity Survey. *Arch Gen Psych.* 1995;52:1048-1060.

2. American Psychiatric Association. *Diagnostic and Statistical Manual of Mental Disorders (DSM-IV).* Fourth edition. Text revision. Washington, DC: American Psychiatric Association; 2000.

3. Dean E. *Shook over Hell: Post-traumatic stress, Vietnam, and the Civil War.* Cambridge, MA: Harvard University Press; 1997.

4. Kulka RA, Schlenger WE, Fairbank JA, et al. Trauma and the Vietnam War generation: report of findings from the National Vietnam Veterans Readjustment Study. New York: Brunner/Mazel; 1990.

5. Kang HK, Natelson BH, Mahan CM, et al. Post-traumatic stress disorder and chronic fatigue syndrome-like illness among Gulf War veterans: a population-based survey of 30,000 veterans. *Am J Epidemiol.* 2003;157:141-148.

6. Taubman-Ben-Ari O, Rabinowitz J, Feldman D, Vaturi R. Post-traumatic stress disorder in primary-care settings: prevalence and physicians' detection. *Psychol Med.* 2001;31:555-560.

7. Brady KT, Killeen TK, Brewerton T, et al. Comorbidity of psychiatric disorders and posttraumatic stress disorder. *J Clin Psychiatry.* 2000;61[Suppl 7]:22-32.

8. Davidson JRT. Pharmacological treatment of acute and chronic stress following trauma. *J Clin Psychiatry.* 2006;67[Suppl 2]:34-39.

9. Ballenger JC, Davidson JR, Lecruibier Y, et al. Consensus statement on posttraumatic stress disorder from the International Consensus Group on Depression and Anxiety. *J Clin Psychiatry.* 2000;61[suppl 5]:60-66.

10. Stein DJ, Davidson J, Seedat S, Beebe K. Paroxetine in the treatment of post-traumatic stress disorder: pooled analysis of placebo-controlled studies. *Expert Opin Pharmacother.* 2003;4:1829-1838.

11. Brady K, Pearlstein T, Asnis GM, et al. Efficacy and safety of sertraline treatment of posttraumatic stress disorder: a randomized controlled trial. *JAMA.* 2000;283:1837-1844.

12. Davidson JR, Rothbaum BO, van der Kolk BA, et al. Multicenter, double-blind comparison of sertraline and placebo in the treatment of posttraumatic stress disorder. *Arch Gen Psychiatry.* 2001;58:485-492.

13. Schoenfeld FB, Marmar CR, Neylan TC. Current concepts in pharmacotherapy of posttraumatic stress disorder. *Psychiatric Serv.* 2004;55:519-531.

14. Londborg PD, Hegel MT, Goldstein S, et al. Sertraline treatment of posttraumatic stress disorder: results of 24 weeks of open-label continuation treatments. *J Clin*

Psychiatry. 2001;62:325-331.

15. Davidson J, Rothbaum BO, Tucker P, et al. Venlafaxine extended release in posttraumatic stress disorder: a sertraline-and placebo-controlled study. *J Clin Psychopharmacol.* 2006;26:259-267.

16. Frank JB, Kosten TR, Giller EL Jr, Dan E. A randomized clinical trial of phenelzine and imipramine for posttraumatic stress disorder. *Am J Psychiatry.* 1988;145:1289-1291.

17. Kosten T, Frank J, Dan E, et al. Pharmacotherapy for posttraumatic stress disorder using phenelzine or imipramine. *J Nerv Ment Dis.* 1991;179:366-370.

18. Davidson K, Kudler H, Smith R, et al. Treatment of posttraumatic stress disorder with amitriptyline or placebo. *Arch Gen Psychiatry.* 1990;47:259-266.

19. Dow B, Kline N. Antidepressant treatment of posttraumatic stress disorder and major depression in veterans. *Ann Clin Psychiatry.* 1997;9:1-5.

20. McRae AL, Brady KT, Mellman TA et al. Comparison of nefazodone and sertraline for the treatment of posttraumatic stress disorder. *Depress Anxiety.* 2004;19:190-196.

21. Mellman TA, David D, Barza L. Nefazodone treatment and dream reports in chronic PTSD. *Depress Anxiety.* 1999;9:146-148.

22. Bartzokis G, Lu PH, Turner J, et al. Adjunctive risperidone in the treatment of combat-related posttraumatic stress disorder. *Biol Psychiatry.* 2005;57:474-479.

23. Monnelly EP, Ciraulo DA, Knapp C, Keane T. Low-dose risperidone as adjunctive therapy for irritable aggression in posttraumatic stress disorder. *J Clin Psychopharmacol.* 2003;23:193-196.

24. Pivac N, Kozaric-Kovacic D, Muck-Seler D. Olanzapine versus fluphenazine in an open trial in patients with psychotic combat-related post-traumatic stress disorder. *Psychopharmacol (Berl.)*2004;175:451-456.

25. Petty F, Brannan S, Casada J, et al. Olanzapine treatment for post-traumatic stress disorder: an open-label study. *Int Clin Psychopharmacol.* 2001;16:331-337.

26. Hamner MB, Deitsch SE, Brodrick PS, et al. Quetiapine treatment in patients with posttraumatic stress disorder: an open trial of adjunctive therapy. *J Clin Psychopharmacol.* 2003;23:15-20.

27. Siddiqui Z, Marcil WA, Bhatia SC, et al. Ziprasidone therapy for post-traumatic stress disorder. *J Psychiatry Neurosci.* 2005;30:430-431.

28. Lambert MT. Aripiprazole in the management of post-traumatic stress disorder symptoms in returning Global War on Terrorism veterans. *Int Clin Psychopharmacol.* 2006;21:185-187.

29. Pivac N, Kozaric-Kovacic D. Pharmacotherapy of treatment-resistant combat-related posttraumatic stress disorder with psychotic features. *Croat Med J.* 2006;47:440-451.

30. American Diabetes Association; American Psychiatric Association; American Association of Clinical Endocrinologists; North American Association for the Study of Obesity. Consensus development conference on antipsychotic drugs and obesity and diabetes. *Diabetes Care.* 2004;27:596-601.

31. Braun P, Greenberg D, et al. Core symptoms of posttraumatic stress disorder

unimproved by alprazolam treatment. *J Clin Psychiatry*. 1990;51:236-238.

32. Mellman TA, Byers PM, Augenstein JS. Pilot evaluation of hypnotic medication during acute traumatic stress response. *J Trauma Stress*. 1998;11:563-569.

33. Gelpin E, Bonne O, Peri T, et al. Treatment of recent trauma survivors with benzodiazepines: a prospective study. *J Clin Psychiatry*. 1996;57:390-394.

34. Yehuda R, Siever LJ, Teicher MH, et al. Plasma norepinephrine and 3-methoxy-4-hydroxyphenylglycol concentrations and severity of depression in combat posttraumatic stress disorder and major depressive disorder. *Biol Psychiatry*. 1998;44:56-63.

35. Pitman RK, Delahanty DL. Conceptually driven pharmacologic approaches to acute trauma. *CNS Spectr*. 2005;10:99-106.

36. Raskind MA, Peskind ER, Kanter ED, et al. Reduction of nightmares and other PTSD symptoms in combat veterans by prazosin: a placebo-controlled study. *Am J Psychiatry*. 2003;160:371-373.

37. Taylor FB, Lowe K, Thompson C, et al. Daytime prazosin reduces psychological distress to trauma specific cues in civilian trauma posttraumatic stress disorder. *Biol Psychiatry*. 2006;59:577-581.

38. Vaiva G, Ducrocq F, Jezequel K, et al. Immediate treatment with propranolol decreases posttraumatic stress disorder two months after trauma. *Biol Psychiatry*. 2003;54:947-949.

39. Pittman RK, Sanders KM, Zusman RM, et al. Pilot study of secondary prevention of posttraumatic stress disorder with propranolol. *Biol Psychiatry*. 2002;15:189-192.

40. Lipper S, Davidson JRT, Grade TA, et al. Preliminary study of carbamazepine in post-traumatic stress disorder. *Psychosomatics*. 1986;27:849-854.

41. Fesler FA. Valproate in combat-related posttraumatic stress disorder. *J Clin Psychiatry*. 1991;52:361-364.

42. Berlant J, van Kammen DP. Open-label topiramate as primary or adjunctive therapy in chronic civilian posttraumatic stress disorder: a preliminary report. *J Clin Psychiatry*. 2002;63:15-20.

43. Hammer MB, Brodrick PS, Labbate LA. Gabapentin in PTSD: a retrospective, clinical series of adjunctive therapy. *Ann Clin Psychiatry*. 2001;13:141-146.

44. Hertzberg MA, Butterfield MI, Feldman ME, et al. A preliminary study of lamotrigine for the treatment of posttraumatic stress disorder. *Biol Psychiatry*. 1999;45:1226-1229.

45. Hoge C, McGurk D, Thomas J, Cox A, Engel C, Castro, C (2008). Mild traumatic brain injury in U.S. soldiers returning from Iraq. New England Journal of Medicine. 358(5):453.

46. Seale K, Bertenthal D, Miner C, Sen S, Marmar C (2007). Bringing the war back home: Mental health disorders among 103 788 US Veterans returning from Iraq and Afghanistan seen at department of veteran affairs facilities. Archives of Internal Medicine. 167:476.

47. Kovach G. Combat's inner cost (2007). Newsweek. 150(19).

48. Roth T. Insomnia: Epidemiology, characteristics, and consequences (2003). Clinical

Cornerstone. 5(3).

49. Figley CR, Nash WR (2007). Combat stress injury: Theory, research, and management. New York, NY: Brunner-Routledge.

50. Anis G, Kohn S, Henderson M, Brown N (2004). SSRIs versus non-SSRIs in post-traumatic stress disorder: an update with recommendations. Drugs. 64:383-404.

51. Wilson JP, Friedman MJ, Lindy JD (2004). Treating psychological trauma & PTSD. New York, NY: The Guilford Press.

52. Hollifield M, Sinclair-Lian N, Warner T, Hammerschlag R (2007). Acupuncture for posttraumatic stress disorder: A randomized controlled pilot trial. The Journal of Nervous and Mental Disease. 195:504-513.

53. Spence DW, Kayumov L, Chen A, Lowe A, Jain U, Katzman M, Shen J, Perelman B, Shapiro C (2004). Acupuncture increases nocturnal melatonin secretion and reduces insomnia and anxiety: A preliminary report. The Journal of Neuropsychiatry and Clinical Neurosciences. 16:19-28.

54. Hernandez-Reif M, Ironson G, Field T, Hurley J, Katz G, Diego M, Weiss S, Fletcher MA, Schanberg S, Kuhn C, Burman I (2004). Breast cancer patients have immune and neuroendocrine functions following massage therapy. Journal of Psychosomatic Research. 57:45-52.

55. Vasterling J, Brewin C (2005). Neuropsychology of PTSD: Biological, cognitive, and clinical perspectives. New York, NY: The Guilford Press.

56. Field T, Hernandez-Reif M, Diego M, Schanberg S, Kuhn C (2005). Cortisol decreases and serotonin and dopamine increase following massage therapy. Inter. J. Neuroscience. 115:1397-1413.

57. Yang CH, Lee BH, Sohn SH (2008). A possible mechanism underlying the effectiveness of acupuncture in the treatment of drug addiction. Evidenced-Based Complementary and Alternative Medicine. 5(3):257-266.

58. Tanielian T, Jaycox L (2008). Invisible Wounds of War: Psychological and cognitive injuries, their consequences, and services to recovery. Arlington, VA: RAND Corporation.

59. Spira, A (2008). Acupuncture: A useful tool for health care in an operational medicine environment. Military Medicine. 173(7):629.

60. Herman J (1997). Trauma and Recovery: The aftermath of violence- from domestic abuse to political terror. New York, NY: Basic Books.

61. Tick E (2005). War and the Soul: Healing our nation's veterans from post-traumatic stress disorder. Wheaton, IL: Quest Books.

62. Yehuda R, Southwick SM, Ma X, et al: Urinary catecholamine excretion and severity of symptoms in PTSD. *J Nerv Men Dis,* 180:321-325, 1992.

63. Yehuda R, Siever L, Teicher MH, et al. Plasma norepinephrine and MHPG concentrations and severity of depression in combat PTSD and major depressive disorder. *Biol Psych,* 44:56-63, 1998.

64. Yehuda R, Southwick SM, Nussbaum G, et al: Low urinary cortisol excretion in patients with PTSD. *J Nerv Ment Dis,* 178:366-309, 1990.

Key References

65. Yehuda R, Boisoneau D, Mason JW, Giller EL: Relationship between lymphocyte glucocorticoid receptor number and urinary-cortisol excretion in mood, anxiety, and psychotic disorder. *Biol Psych,* 34:18-25, 1993.

66. Yehuda R, Kahana B, Binder-Brynes K, et al: Low urinary cortisol excretion in Holocaust survivors with posttraumatic stress disorder. *Am J Psychiatry,* 152:982-986, 1995.

67. Kellner M, Baker D, Yehuda R: Salivary cortisol in Desert Storm returnees. *Biol Psych,* 41: 849-850, 1997.

68. Goenjian AK, Yehuda R, Pynoos RS, et al. Basal cortisol and dexamethasone suppression of cortisol among adolescents after the 1988 earthquake in Armenia. *Am J Psychiatry,* 153: 929-934, 1996.

69. Stein MB, Yehuda R, Koverola C, Hanna C: HPA Axis functioning in adult Women who report experiencing severe childhood sexual abuse, *Biol Psychiatry,* 42:680-686, 1997.

70. Resnick HS, Yehuda R, Foy DW, Pitman R: Effect of prior trauma on acute hormonal response to rape. *Am J Psychiatry,* 152:1675-1677, 1995.

71. Yehuda R, Shalev AY, McFarlane AC. Predicting the development of posttraumatic stress disorder from the acute response to a traumatic event. *Biol Psych,* 44:1305-1313, 1998.

72. Yehuda R, Southwick SM, Krystal JM, et al: Enhanced suppression of cortisol following dexamethasone administration in combat veterans with PTSD and major depressive disorder. *Am J Psychiatry,* 150:83-86, 1993.

73. Yehuda R, Boisoneau D, Lowy MT, Giller EL: Dose-response changes in plasma cortisol and lymphocyte glucocorticoid receptors following dexamethasone administration in combat veterans with and without PTSD. *Arch of Gen Psych,* 52:583-593, 1995.

74. Goenjian AK, Yehuda R, Pynoos RS, et al. Basal cortisol and dexamethasone suppression of cortisol among adolescents after the 1988 earthquake in Armenia. *Am J Psychiatry,* 153: 929-934, 1996.

75. Yehuda R, Levengood RA, Schmeidler RA, et al: Increased pituitary activation following metyrapone administration in PTSD. *Psychoneuroendocrinology,* 21: 1-16, 1996.

76. Yehuda R, Resnick HS, Schmiedler H, et al. Predictors of cortisol and MHPG responses in the acute aftermath of rape. *Biol Psych,* 43:855-859, 1998.

77. Yehuda R. Parental PTSD as a Risk Factor for PTSD, in Yehuda (Ed *Risk Factors for Posttraumatic Stress Disorder).* Progress in Psychiatry Series, American Psychiatric Association, Inc., 1999.

78. Li Zhong-yi, He Fangrui. Integrated Chinese and Western medicine Treatment of PTSD. *Journal of Clinical Psychosomatic Disease,* 2003, 9(1):19-20.

79. Wang Wei-dong. Methods and Applications Required for Preventive TCM Psychology on the Post-earthquake Psychological Crisis. *Journal of Traditional Chinese Medicine,* 2008, 49(11):1034-1036.

80. Wang Mi-qu, Li Wei-song, and Cai Xin, etc. Bipolar Evaluation of Variables in Post-earthquake DM patients. *Liaoning Journal of Traditional Chinese Medicine,* 2009, 36(3):321-323.

81. Wang Yu and Hu You-ping Acupuncture Treatment of 69 PTSD Cases caused by Earthquake. *Henan Journal of Traditional Chinese Medicine,* 2009, 29(3):291.

82. Yuan Xiu-li, Liu Chi, and Lai Ren. Acupuncture Treatment in 34 Cases of PTSD. *Chinese Acupuncture and Moxibustion,* 2009, 29(3):234.

83. Blanchard MS, Eisen SA, Alpern R, Karlinsky J, Toomey R, Reda DJ, Murphy FM, Jackson LW, Kang HK. Chronic multisymptom illness complex in Gulf War I veterans 10 after 10 years. Am J Epidemiol. 2006 Jan 1;163(1):66-75. Epub 2005 Nov 17.

84. Research Advisory Committee on Gulf War Veterans' Illnesses. Gulf War Illness and the Health of Gulf War Veterans: Scientific Findings and Recommendations. Washington, D.C: U.S. Government Printing Office, November 2008. (www1.va.gov/RAC-GWVI/).

85. Rosof B, Hernandez L, Institute of Medicine, Eds. Gulf War Veterans: Treating Symptoms and Syndromes. Washington, DC: National Academy Press, 2001.

86. Liu Jia-qiang, Wang Mi-qu. Combination of TCM psychology and modern psychology. Chinese Archives of Traditional Chinese Medicine. 2008, 26 (3):530-531.

87. Sun Li-yun, Xu Xu-ying "Nei Jing" and medical psychology. Beijing Journal of Traditional Chinese Medicine. 2006, 25 (1): 22 - 23.

88. Yan Shi-Yun. Doctrines of various historical schools in TCM. Beijing: China Press of Traditional Chinese Medicine. 2003. p. 109–110.

89. Ren Ying-qiu. Doctrines of various historical schools in TCM. Shanghai: Shanghai Science and Technology Press; 1998. p. 561.

90. Jiang Yong. TCM behavioral medicine. Beijing: China Press of Traditional Chinese Medicine; 2007. p. 32-35.

91. Wang Mi-qu. TCM psychology. Tianjin: Tianjin Science and Technology Press; 1985. p.174.

92. American Psychiatric Association: *Diagnostic and Statistical Manual of Mental Disorders, Fourth Edition, Revised.* Washington, DC, American Psychiatric Association, 2000.

93. Shin LM, Rauch SL, Pitman RK. Amygdala, medial prefrontal cortex, and hippocampal function in PTSD. *Ann N Y Acad Sci.* 2006; 1071:67-79.

94. de Kloet CS, Vermetten E, Geuze E, et al. Assessment of HPA-axis function in posttraumatic stress disorder: pharmacological and non-pharmacological challenge tests, a review. J Psychiatr Res. 2006;40(6):550-67.

95. Geracioti TD Jr, Baker DG, Kasckow JW, et al. Effects of trauma-related audiovisual stimulation on cerebrospinal fluid norepinephrine and corticotropin-releasing hormone concentrations in post-traumatic stress disorder. *Psychoneuroendocrinology.* 2008;33(4):416-24.

96. Geracioti TD Jr, Baker DG, Ekhator NN, et al. CSF Norepinephrine Concentrations in Posttraumatic Stress Disorder. *Am J Psychiatry.* 2001; 158:1227-1230.

97. Inoue T, Tsuchiya K, Koyama T. Regional changes in dopamine and serotonin activation with various intensity of physical and psychological stress in the rat brain. *Pharmacol Biochem Behav* 1994; 49(4): 911-920.

98. Neumeister, Alexander. What Role Does Serotonin Play in PTSD. Psychiatric Times 2006 April; 23(4) http://pychiatrictimes.com /showArticle.jhtml?articleId= 186700462 (accessed September 19, 2009).

99. Sadock Benjamin J, Sadock Virgina A. Theories of Personality and Psychopathology, Posttraumatic Stress Disorder and Acute Stress Disorder. *Synopsis of Psychiatry, Behavioral Science/Clinical Psychiatry.* Ninth Edition. Philadelphia: Lippincott Williams &Wilkins Press. 2003; pp. 193-210, 623-642.

100. McWilliams Nancy. Secondary (Higher-Order) Defensive Processes" and "Dissociative Personalities *Psychoanalytic Diagnosis: Understanding Personality Process in the Clinical Process.* New York: The Guilford Press, 1994; pp. 40, 117-167 and 323-347.

101. Leahy Robert L, McGinn Lata K, Busch Fredic N, Milrod Barbara L. . Anxiety Disorders. In: Gabbard GO, Beck JS, Holmes J, ed. *Oxford Textbook of Psychotherapy.* Oxford: The Oxford Press, 2005; pp. 137-161.

102. Foa EB, Rothbaum BO, Molnar C. "Cognitive-behavioral therapy of post traumatic stress disorder" In: Friedman MJ, Chamey DS, Deutch AY, ed. *Neurobiological and clinical consequences of stress: from normal adaptation to posttraumatic stress disorder.* Philadelphia, PA: Raven Press, 1995; pp. 483-94.

103. Brown Daniel P, Hammond Corydon D, Scheflin Alan W. *Memory, Trauma Treatment, and the Law.* New York: Norton Press; 1998.

104. Myss Caroline. *Anatomy of the Spirit: The Seven Stages of Power and Healing.* New York: Three Rivers Press; 1996.

105. Hui KK, Liu J, Makris N, et al. Acupuncture Modulates the Limbic System and Subcortical Gray Structures of the Human Brain: Evidence from fMRI Studies in Normal Subjects. *Human Brain Mapping,* 2000; 9:13-25.

106. Hui KK, Liu J, Marina O, et al. The integrated response of the human cerebro-cerebellar and limbic systems to acupuncture stimulation at ST 36 as evidence by fMRI. *Neuro Image.* 2005; 27: 479-496.

107. Lipton, Bruce H. Ph. D. *The Biology of Belief.* Carlsbad, CA: Hay House Inc.; 2005.

108. Edward Tick. *War and the Soul,* Quest Books. Wheaton: The Theosophical Publishing House; 2005. p.16.

109. Bryant, RA, & Harvey, AG. Acute Stress reponse: A comparison of head injured and non-head injured patients. Psychological Medicine, 1995(25): 869-874.

110. Rattock, J. & Ross B. Post-traumatic stress disorder in traumatically head injured. Journal of Clinical and Experimental Neuropsychology (Abstract), 1993(6): 243.

111. Hickling, EJ et al. Traumatic brain injury and posttraumatic stress disorder: A preliminary investigation of neuropsychological test results in PTSD secondary to motor vehicle accidents. *Brain Injury,* 1998(12): 265-274.

Index

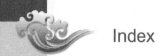

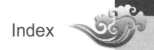

emperor heart-supplementing elixir), 30, 105
tinnitus, 19, 23, 29
traumatic brain injury (TBI), 124
tricyclic antidepressants (TCAs), 55

W

Wēn Dǎn Tāng (Gallbladder-Warming Decoction), 24

X

Xiāo Yáo Sǎn (Rambling Powder), 117
Xuán Fù Dài Zhě Tāng (Inula and
Hematite Decoction), 19

Y

yin fire, 14, 77
yìn táng (EX-HN3), 32, 60, 72

图书在版编目（CIP）数据

中西医结合治疗创伤后应激障碍（英文）/ Joe C. Chang,
汪卫东, 江泳主编. —北京: 人民卫生出版社, 2010.3
ISBN 978-7-117-12358-7

Ⅰ. ①中⋯ Ⅱ. ①J⋯ ②汪⋯ ③江⋯ Ⅲ. ①创伤—心理
应激—研究—英文 Ⅳ. ①R641

中国版本图书馆CIP数据核字（2009）第244406号

门户网：www.pmph.com	出版物查询、网上书店
卫人网：www.ipmph.com	护士、医师、药师、中医师、卫生资格考试培训

中西医结合治疗创伤后应激障碍（英文）

主　　编：Joe C. Chang，汪卫东，江泳
出版发行：人民卫生出版社（+8610-5978 7399）
地　　址：中国北京市朝阳区潘家园南里19号
邮　　编：100021
E - mail：pmph @ pmph.com
发　　行：pmphsales @ gmail.com
购书热线：+8610-5978 7399/5978 7338（电话及传真）
开　　本：787×1092　1/16
版　　次：2010年3月第1版　2010年3月第1版第1次印刷
标准书号：ISBN 978-7-117-12358-7/R·12359